The State of Podiatric Science

Editor

ANDREW J. MEYR

CLINICS IN PODIATRIC MEDICINE AND SURGERY

www.podiatric.theclinics.com

Consulting Editor
THOMAS J. CHANG

April 2024 • Volume 41 • Number 2

ELSEVIER

1600 John F. Kennedy Boulevard • Suite 1800 • Philadelphia, Pennsylvania, 19103-2899

http://www.theclinics.com

CLINICS IN PODIATRIC MEDICINE AND SURGERY Volume 41, Number 2
April 2024 ISSN 0891-8422, ISBN-13: 978-0-443-12985-8

Editor: Megan Ashdown
Developmental Editor: Anita Chamoli

Clinics in Podiatric Medicine and Surgery (ISSN 0891-8422) is published quarterly by Elsevier Inc., 360 Park Avenue South, New York, NY 10010-1710. Months of issue are January, April, July, and October. Business and Editorial Offices: 1600 John F. Kennedy Blvd., Ste. 1800, Philadelphia, PA 19103-2899. Customer Service Office: 3251 Riverport Lane, Maryland Heights, MO 63043. Periodicals postage paid at New York, NY and additional mailing offices. Subscription prices are $332.00 per year for US individuals, $100.00 per year for US students and residents, $417.00 per year for Canadian individuals, $505.00 for international individuals, $100.00 per year for Canadian students/residents, and $220.00 per year for foreign students/residents. For institutional access pricing please contact Customer Service via the contact information below. To receive student/resident rate, orders must be accompanied by name of affiliated institution, date of term, and the *signature* of program/residency coordinator on institution letterhead. Orders will be billed at individual rate until proof of status is received. Foreign air speed delivery is included in all *Clinics* subscription prices. All prices are subject to change without notice. POSTMASTER: Send address changes to *Clinics in Podiatric Medicine and Surgery*, Elsevier Health Sciences Division, Subscription Customer Service, 3251 Riverport Lane, Maryland Heights, MO 63043. **Customer Service: 1-800-654-2452 (US). From outside of the US, call 314-447-8871. Fax: 314-447-8029. E-mail: JournalsCustomerService-usa@elsevier.com (for print support); JournalsOnline-Support-usa@elsevier.com (for online support).**

Reprints. For copies of 100 or more of articles in this publication, please contact the Commercial Reprints Department, Elsevier Inc., 360 Park Avenue South, New York, NY 10010-1710. Tel.: 212-633-3874; Fax: 212-633-3820; E-mail: reprints@elsevier.com.

Clinics in Podiatric Medicine and Surgery is covered in *MEDLINE/PubMed (Index Medicus)* and *EMBASE/Excerpta Medica*.

Contributors

CONSULTING EDITOR

THOMAS J. CHANG, DPM
Clinical Professor and Past Chairman, Department of Podiatric Surgery, CCPM, Faculty,
The Podiatry Institute, Sonoma County Orthopedic & Podiatric Specialists, Santa Rosa,
California

EDITOR

ANDREW J. MEYR, DPM, FACFAS
Professor, Department of Surgery, Temple University School of Podiatric Medicine,
Philadelphia, Pennsylvania

AUTHORS

MONICA R. AGARWAL, DPM, FACFAS
Clinical Assistant Professor, Department of Medicine, School of Podiatric Medicine, The
University of Texas Rio Grande Valley, Edinburg, Texas

RACHEL H. ALBRIGHT, DPM, MPH, FACFAS
Podiatrist, Foot and Ankle Surgery, Podiatry, Department of Surgery, Stamford Health
Medical Group, Stamford, Connecticut

ELIZABETH ANSERT, MA, DPM, MBA, AACFAS
Fellow, Department of Plastic Surgery, University of Texas Southwestern Diabetic and
Limb Salvage, The University of Texas Southwestern Medical Center, Dallas, Texas

DAVID G. ARMSTRONG, DPM, MD, PhD
Director, Professor of Surgery, Keck School of Medicine of USC, Southwestern Academic
Limb Salvage Alliance, Los Angeles, California

DAVID AUNGST, DPM, FACFAS
Health Science Assistant Clinical Professor, Department of Surgery, David Geffen School
of Medicine, University of California, Los Angeles, Los Angeles, California

JARRETT D. CAIN, DPM
Associate Professor, Department of Orthopedic Surgery, University of Pittsburgh School
of Medicine, University of Pittsburgh Physicians, Pittsburgh, Pennsylvania

ALAN CATANZARITI, DPM, FACFAS
Attending Surgeon, Department of Orthopedics, West Penn Hospital Foot and Ankle
Surgery, Allegheny Health Network, Pittsburgh, Pennsylvania

NICOLE K. CATES, DPM, AACFAS
Fellowship Trained Foot and Ankle Surgeon, Hand and Microsurgery Medical Group,
San Francisco, California

EMILY A. COOK, DPM, MPH, CPH
Director of Resident Training, Division of Podiatric Surgery, Department of Surgery, Mount Auburn Hospital, Cambridge, Massachusetts; Harvard Medical School, Boston, Massachusetts

JEREMY J. COOK, DPM, MPH, CPH
Director of Research, Division of Podiatric Surgery, Department of Surgery, Mount Auburn Hospital, Cambridge, Massachusetts; Assistant Professor of Surgery, Harvard Medical School, Boston, Massachusetts

ANDREW CRISOLOGO, DPM, AACFAS
Assistant Professor, Attending Physician, Department of Plastic Surgery, The University of Texas Southwestern Medical Center, Dallas, Texas

ADAM E. FLEISCHER, DPM, MPH, FACFAS
Director, Podiatric Medicine and Surgery Residency Program, Advocate Illinois Masonic Medical Center/RFUMS, Director of Research, Weil Foot and Ankle Institute, Chicago, Illinois; Professor, Department of Podiatric Medicine and Surgery, Rosalind Franklin University of Medicine and Science (RFUMS), North Chicago, Illinois

SEAN GRAMBART, DPM, FACFAS
Assistant Dean for Clinical Affairs, Des Moines University College of Podiatric Medicine and Surgery, Des Moines, Iowa

JESSICA JASWAL, DPM, MS, PGY3
Department of Surgery, University of California, Los Angeles, Los Angeles, California

ROBERT JOSEPH, DPM, PhD, FACFAS
Gainesville, Florida

WARREN S. JOSEPH, DPM, FIDSA
Adjunct Clinical Professor, Arizona College of Podiatric Medicine, Midwestern University, Glendale, Arizona; Editor, *Journal of the American Podiatric Medical Association*, Hatboro, Pennsylvania

DANIEL C. JUPITER, PhD
Associate Professor, Departments of Biostatistics and Data Science, and Orthopaedic Surgery and Rehabilitation, The University of Texas Medical Branch, Galveston, Texas

PAUL J. KIM, MS, DPM, FACFAS
Professor, Attending Physician, Department of Plastic Surgery, The University of Texas Southwestern Medical Center, Dallas, Texas

ERIN E. KLEIN, DPM, MS
Fellowship Trained Foot and Ankle Surgeon, Associate Director of Research, Weil Foot and Ankle Institute, Mount Prospect, Dr William M Scholl College of Podiatric; Clinical Instructor, Medicine at Rosalind Franklin University of Medicine and Science, North Chicago, Illinois

ADAM S. LANDSMAN, DPM, PhD
Assistant Professor, Division of Podiatric Surgery, Department of Orthopedic Surgery, Massachusetts General Hospital, Harvard Medical School, Boston, Massachusetts

EMILY LOBOS, DPM
Resident Physician, Division of Foot and Ankle Surgery, Department of Orthopedics, West Penn Hospital, Pittsburgh, Pennsylvania

DONALD SCOT MALAY, DPM, MSCE, FACFAS
Staff Surgeon and Director of Podiatric Research, Penn Presbyterian Medical Center, Philadelphia, Pennsylvania; Editor Emeritus, *The Journal of Foot and Ankle Surgery*

RYAN McMILLEN, DPM, FACFAS
Attending Surgeon, Department of Orthopedics, West Penn Hospital Foot and Ankle Surgery, Allegheny Health Network, Pittsburgh, Pennsylvania

ANDREW J. MEYR, DPM, FACFAS
Professor, Department of Surgery, Temple University School of Podiatric Medicine, Philadelphia, Pennsylvania

AKSONE NOUVONG, DPM, FACFAS
Health Science Clinical Professor, Department of Surgery, David Geffen School of Medicine, University of California, Los Angeles, Los Angeles, California

JASON PIRIANO, DPM, MS, FACFAS
Associate Professor, Chief of Foot and Ankle Surgery, Director of Residency Training and Podiatric Surgery, Department of Orthopaedics and Rehabilitation, University of Florida, College of Medicine-Jacksonville, Jacksonville, Florida

TYLER RODERICKS, DPM
Chief Resident, Division of Podiatric Surgery, Department of Surgery, Mount Auburn Hospital, Cambridge, Massachusetts; Clinical Fellow in Surgery, Harvard Medical School, Boston, Massachusetts

THOMAS S. ROUKIS, DPM, PhD, FACFAS
Clinical Professor, Associate Director Residency Training-Podiatric Surgery, Department of Orthopaedics and Rehabilitation, University of Florida, College of Medicine-Jacksonville, Jacksonville, Florida

LAURA E. SANSOSTI, DPM, FACFAS
Associate Professor, Departments of Surgery and Biomechanics, Temple University School of Podiatric Medicine, Philadelphia, Pennsylvania

NAOHIRO SHIBUYA, DPM, MS, FACFAS
Clinical Professor of Medicine, School of Podiatric Medicine, The University of Texas Rio Grande Valley, Edinburg, Texas

JOHN STEINBERG, DPM
Attending Physician, Department of Plastic Surgery, MedStar Georgetown University Hospital, Washington, DC

CRAIG VERDIN, DPM
Fellow, Department of Plastic Surgery, MedStar Georgetown University Hospital, Washington, DC

TRACEY VLAHOVIC, DPM
Professor, Department of Medicine, Temple University School of Podiatric Medicine, Philadelphia, Pennsylvania

CAITLIN ZARICK, DPM
Attending Physician, Department of Plastic Surgery, MedStar Georgetown University Hospital, Washington, DC

Contents

Foreword: The State of Podiatric Science   xiii

Thomas J. Chang

Preface   xv

Andrew J. Meyr

Introduction   xvii

David G. Armstrong

A Study Never *Proves* Anything: Contemporary Interpretation of the Levels of Clinical Evidence and Statistical Significance   215

Andrew J. Meyr

Critical analysis of the medical literature and an evidence-based approach to clinical practice and medical decision-making is of vital importance in contemporary podiatric practice. This article reviews the levels of clinical evidence and their application within this paradigm. This includes determining which level of evidence is most appropriate for a given methodology, as well as an appreciation of inherent limitations within each level of evidence. The article concludes with a discussion on the difference between statistical significance and clinical significance.

Basic Statistics, Statistical Design, and Critical Analysis of Statistics for Surgeons   223

Andrew J. Meyr and Daniel Jupiter

Statistics is a set of tools used in medical decision-making no different than how a scalpel or a sagittal saw is used in the operating room. No foot and ankle surgeon is born with the inherent ability to perform, understand, and critically interpret them. Instead, it requires training and practice throughout the course of a career in medicine to develop a working proficiency. This article reviews the basic indications and interpretation of common descriptive and comparative statistical tests in the podiatric literature. Additionally, the concept of which tests are most appropriate for which investigational methodologies is introduced.

Incorporating Research into a Busy Clinical Practice: A Practical Approach   233

Erin E. Klein

Treating patients in clinic can be busy and stressful; however, utilization of well-planned strategic workflows that include the proper information for research studies can result in daily prospective data collection that will be subsequently amenable to retrospective analysis.

Navigating Institutional Review Boards   239

Elizabeth Ansert, Nicole K. Cates, Andrew Crisologo, and Paul J. Kim

> Obtaining institutional review board (IRB) approval can be an overwhelming task, especially for new researchers. IRB approval can require many documents and steps. It is important to start the submission early, have patience throughout the process, and determine what can help expedite the process. Research cannot begin without IRB approval, which is necessary when working with human subjects. Ultimately, the researchers and IRB have the same goal of enabling good research with minimal subject risk. The goal of this article is to give an overview of the IRB for practitioners performing research in podiatric medicine and surgery.

Grants and Funding in Podiatric Science   247

Aksone Nouvong, Jessica Jaswal, and David Aungst

> Evidence-based research is essential to improving podiatric medicine and surgery; however, there are many barriers to conducting research, with a major limitation being lack of research funding. There are various grants and funding sources available to podiatric surgeon scientists, but navigating through the resources can be daunting. In this article, we provide a framework for grant writing and funding opportunities for podiatric surgeons to consider.

A New Paradigm in Foot and Ankle Outcomes?: Away From Radiographs and Toward Patient-Centered Outcomes   259

Naohiro Shibuya, Monica R. Agarwal, and Daniel C. Jupiter

> Having reasonable outcome measures is essential to unbiased research. For years, provider-measured outcomes have been valued as they are more objective and convenient for investigators. However, with the popularity of patient-centered medical care delivery, patient-reported outcome measures are appropriately becoming more popular in foot and ankle research.

Effective Case Reports and Small Case Series   269

Jason Piriano and Thomas S. Roukis

> Once the mainstay of scientific journals, in the age of evidence-based medicine, case reports and small series are now considered to represent a lower hierarchy in the medical decision-making process. However, case reports and small series represent the culmination of the time-honored traditional medical education teaching method with the descriptive case presentation. Despite being infrequently cited as references, case reports and small series still offer important contributions to patient care. The authors present a review of the strengths and weaknesses of case reports and small series and discuss ways to incorporate this form of literature into structured medical education.

Critical Analysis of Retrospective Study Designs: Cohort and Case Series   273

Emily Lobos, Alan Catanzariti, and Ryan McMillen

> Retrospective studies represent an often used research methodology in the podiatric scientific literature, with cohort studies and case series being

two of the most prevalent designs. Choosing a retrospective method is often dependent on multiple factors, two of the most important being details of the research question to be explored and the sample size that can be acquired. When analyzing literature, a reader must understand how retrospective studies work to critically examine the methods, results, and discussions to determine if the conclusion is reasonable and might be applied to clinical practice.

Prospective Surgical Cohort Analysis   281

Adam E. Fleischer and Rachel H. Albright

A well-conducted prospective cohort study has the potential to change the way in which surgeons practice. However, not all are equal. In this article, we provide many of the tools needed to critically appraise this powerful study design. We advocate for using a 3-step approach that centers on understanding the study's generalizability, results, and validity. We illustrate how this process is applied into practice regularly at our hospital section's journal club sessions.

Narrative Review to Meta-Analysis: A Cookbook Approach to Evidence Synthesis in Surgical Research   291

Jeremy J. Cook, Tyler Rodericks, and Emily A. Cook

Evidence synthesis is a complex approach to research that can consolidate the current understanding of a particular topic from various sources. A design hierarchy based upon reliability is described in detail. Methodology is described explicitly to provide readers with a foundation for performing and understanding published evidence synthesis. Resources that detail access to the comprehensive database are presented and explained. Special care is taken to discuss appraisal of studies prior to analysis.

A Primer on Cost-Effectiveness Analysis   313

Rachel H. Albright and Adam E. Fleischer

A cost-effectiveness analysis (CEA) is a type of health economics model that uses a systematic approach to simplify the complexities that exist in health-care decision-making. A CEA aids in medical decision-making by considering both the costs of a treatment and how effective that treatment is for at least 2 competing strategies. This article reviews major concepts of CEA including results interpretation, key attributes of CEA that make it differ from cost analysis, uncertainty surrounding analysis, and how/why CEA is an important contributor to the medical literature.

Unique Challenges in Diabetic Foot Science   323

Craig Verdin, Caitlin Zarick, and John Steinberg

In the past 30 years, there has been a rapid influx of information pertaining to the diabetic foot (DF) coming from numerous directions and sources. This article discusses the current state of the DF literature and challenges it presents to clinicians with its associated increase in knowledge on their derivations, complications, and interventions. Further, we attempt to provide tips on how to navigate and criticize the current literature to encourage and maximize positive outcomes in this challenging patient population.

Special Considerations in Podiatric Science: Translational Research, Cadavers, Gait Analysis, Dermatology, and Databases   333

Jarrett D. Cain, Tracey Vlahovic, and Andrew J. Meyr

The objective of this article is to provide a brief overview of the critical analysis and design of unique and perhaps less common methodologies in podiatric science. These include basic science translational designs, cadaveric investigations, gait analyses, dermatologic studies, and database analysis. The relative advantages, disadvantages, and inherent limitations are reviewed with an intention to improve the interpretation of results and advance future foot and ankle scientific endeavors.

Working with Industry   343

Adam S. Landsman

In 1992, I completed a 9-year dual-degree program where I received both my DPM degree and a PhD in Bioengineering. Upon my graduation, it was apparent that "Industry" had an interest in me. Sponsored research and consulting opportunities where readily available, and I had to learn very quickly to sort the scientific from the sham, and the clinically worthwhile from the worthless. Partnering with Industry has provided me with another avenue to advance my profession, while helping to develop new treatment options that can potentially help many more patients then just the ones I see in my office.

Effective Manuscript Preparation and Submission   351

Donald Scot Malay

Authors have a wide range of journals to which they can submit their report for consideration for publication. One key to getting the journal editors to accept a report is that the manuscript is properly organized and in compliance with the journal's Guide for Authors. For this reason, the single most important undertaking that an author can do before submission is read the journal's Guide for Authors and make sure that the report meets the journal's requirements for publication. If the subject matter is interesting and scientifically rigorous, then a well-written manuscript that complies with the journal's requirements will likely cruise through the peer review process and get accepted for publication. With this in mind, we now break down the elements of a report of original research and describe useful details that enhance the manuscript and leave little to revise.

The Peer Review System: A Journal Editor's 30-Year Perspective   359

Warren S. Joseph

The peer review system has become the standard by which scientific articles are refereed. Unfortunately, even from its beginnings in the mid-1800s it has been fraught with difficulties. Potential reviewers are volunteers who may be inundated with requests to review yet these reviews take considerable time and effort. There is little motivation to complete a review causing significant delays in the publication process. There may be biases unintentionally built into the system between reviewers, authors, editors, and journals. Attempts to overcome these biases by various blinding schemes have been met with limited success. Finally, the recent advent of Artificial Intelligence has the potential to completely upend the system, for good or bad.

Teaching Science to the Next Generation 367

Laura E. Sansosti, Robert Joseph, and Sean Grambart

Teaching science to the next generation begins with foundations laid in podiatric medical school. Interest and immersion in research continues to develop through residency as trainees prepare for cases, participate in journal clubs, present posters and articles, and attend conferences. Having adequate training is essential to production of quality research. Although challenges and barriers exist, numerous resources are available at all levels of practice to guide those who are interested in contributing to the body of literature that supports the profession. Ensuring a robust pipeline of future clinician scientists is critical to the future of the profession.

CLINICS IN PODIATRIC MEDICINE AND SURGERY

FORTHCOMING ISSUES

July 2024
Current Concepts in Foot and Ankle Trauma
J. Randolph Clements and Mark Hofbauer, *Editors*

October 2024
Minimal Incision Surgery
Neal M. Blitz, *Editor*

January 2025
Basic Principles of External Fixation
Guido LaPorta, *Editor*

RECENT ISSUES

January 2024
The Kaiser Permanente Podiatry Experience: Lessons Learned in Foot and Ankle Surgery
Christy Marie King, *Editor*

October 2023
Updates in Foot and Ankle Arthritis
Jeffrey E. McAlister, *Editor*

July 2023
Arthroscopy of the Foot and Ankle
Laurence Rubin, *Editor*

SERIES OF RELATED INTEREST

Orthopedic Clinics
https://www.orthopedic.theclinics.com/
Clinics in Sports Medicine
https://www.sportsmed.theclinics.com/
Foot and Ankle Clinics
https://www.foot.theclinics.com/
Physical Medicine and Rehabilitation Clinics
https://www.pmr.theclinics.com/

THE CLINICS ARE AVAILABLE ONLINE!
Access your subscription at:
www.theclinics.com

Foreword

The State of Podiatric Science

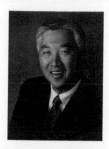

Thomas J. Chang, DPM
Consulting Editor

I am excited to introduce this issue on the "Science" of Podiatric Medicine and Surgery. Being a good scientist does not always come naturally for Clinicians in private practice. Much of our true experience and decisions are based on anecdotal observations through our career. The N = 1 perspective of carefully evaluating and providing individualized treatment for each patient still is vitally important in a successful practice. But times are changing. Patient and outcomes data now dictate many aspects of how we practice health care, with prescribing medications, procedure authorizations, and insurance reimbursements to name a few.

Our profession has embraced this rapid growth and is well positioned for the future.

I remember first hearing about the DPM/PhD program being offered at Pennsylvania College of Podiatric Medicine (PCPM) in 1986, and Dr Adam Landsman was the first candidate accepted into this dual-degree offering. Even then, many of the schools were actively invested in clinical research, and Gait Analysis labs were on the upswing. Journal clubs often discussed how to critically evaluate and grade the quality of published medical literature.

I applaud the work of our journal's editors during this time. Drs Warren Joseph, Lowell Weil Sr., Jack Schuberth, and Scot Malay have brought the level of our peer-reviewed publications on par with many of the top medical journals in the world.

I am grateful to Dr Andrew Meyr for his insight in bringing relevant topics and leading experts into this issue. His passion in sharing his knowledge so we can all better understand the scientific process is well illustrated here. This important work, which occurs within our national organizations and educational institutions, is remarkable, and we are all better for it.

Clin Podiatr Med Surg 41 (2024) xiii–xiv
https://doi.org/10.1016/j.cpm.2023.12.001
0891-8422/24/© 2023 Published by Elsevier Inc.

podiatric.theclinics.com

Best wishes in the New Year.

Thomas J. Chang, DPM
Sonoma County Orthopedic/
Podiatric Specialists
3536 Mendocino Avenue, Suite 300B
Santa Rosa, CA 95403, USA

E-mail address:
thomaschang14@comcast.net

Preface

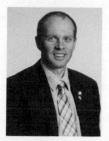

Andrew J. Meyr, DPM, FACFAS
Editor

It is both a privilege and an honor to edit this issue of *Clinics in Podiatric Medicine and Surgery* on the topic of "science" in podiatric medicine and surgery. And to be perfectly candid, it was organized from a position of introspection and pride on my part when considering the importance of science within our profession. My very first experience with the medical literature and my very first PubMed citation was from *Clinics in Podiatric Medicine and Surgery* on the topic of "Pain Management" in July of 2008. Back then, I was an admittedly dopey resident at Inova Fairfax Hospital, and almost certainly in over my head! But I had a determination to help produce something that I believed strongly would be of benefit for our profession in an area that was (at the time...) not of contemporary focus in terms of formal medical education. Fast-forward 15 years, and I am now a Professor in the Department of Surgery at the Temple University of Podiatric Medicine and proud to contribute to many of our profession's leading national organizations and journals.

I can appreciate that some readers might approach this issue with a bit of trepidation. On the surface, the concept of "science" might not seem overly clinical or applicable to daily practice. Please have confidence that I have attempted to both design the topics and challenge the authors to be as practical as possible with their material. We live in an evidence-based world, and this issue aims to bring these concepts as directly as possible to readers in a tangible way:

- For students, we hope to ignite an interest in participation with the scientific process and supplement your medical school education by covering as many concepts as possible as outlined in the AACPM Council of Faculties Curricular Guide.
- For residents and fellows, we hope to provide the groundwork for your instruction and involvement in research methodology as required by the Council on Podiatric Medical Education and American College of Foot and Ankle Surgeons, respectfully.
- For practicing physicians, we hope to continue your academic and scientific growth while feeling confident in your ability to bring the best possible and most contemporary interventions to your patients.

Clin Podiatr Med Surg 41 (2024) xv–xvi
https://doi.org/10.1016/j.cpm.2023.07.002
0891-8422/24/© 2023 Published by Elsevier Inc.

podiatric.theclinics.com

I want to thank the contributing authors for sharing their time, expertise, passion, and practical professional experiences for this issue. I am proud to know, work with, and learn from you all.

I am also grateful to and want to thank Dr David Armstrong, arguably the leading podiatric surgeon-scientist of our profession, for providing the foreword to this issue of *Clinics in Podiatric Medicine and Surgery*.

Andrew J. Meyr, DPM, FACFAS
Department of Surgery
Temple University School of Podiatric Medicine
148 North 8th Street
Philadelphia, PA 19107, USA

E-mail address:
ajmeyr@gmail.com

Introduction

It is with distinct enthusiasm that I introduce this issue of *Clinics in Podiatric Medicine and Surgery* on the important topic of "The State of Podiatric Science." Science is, after all, the engine that fuels the evolution and growth of our specialty.

As we explore the current landscape of podiatric science, I encourage you to approach the content with an open mind and a curious heart, pondering ways in which you might contribute to our shared body of knowledge. We are the stewards of this specialty, and it is our collective responsibility to shape its trajectory, its impact, and its future.

I want to express my sincere gratitude to Dr Meyr for his tireless work in bringing this issue together. Our specialty thrives thanks to the dedication and efforts of individuals like him.

Let us remember the importance of our collective pursuit. Here's to expanding our knowledge, to pushing the boundaries of podiatric medicine and surgery, and, most importantly, to helping people move through the world a little better.

Yours very truly,

David G. Armstrong, DPM, MD, PhD
Keck School of Medicine of USC
1975 Zonal Avenue
Los Angeles, CA 90033, USA

E-mail address:
armstrong@usa.net

Clin Podiatr Med Surg 41 (2024) xvii
https://doi.org/10.1016/j.cpm.2023.07.011
0891-8422/24/© 2023 Published by Elsevier Inc.

A Study Never *Proves* Anything
Contemporary Interpretation of the Levels of Clinical Evidence and Statistical Significance

Andrew J. Meyr, DPM

KEYWORDS

- Level of evidence • Evidence based • Clinical significance • Retrospective
- Prospective • Randomized controlled trial

KEY POINTS

- Critical analysis of the medical literature requires subjective evaluation of objective methodology and results.
- All published studies have limitations. Critical analysis of the medical literature involves interpreting the results of investigations in light of these limitations and not rejecting the results because of them.
- Developing a clinical hypothesis and asking appropriate clinical questions is an important first step in determining the level of clinical evidence.
- Most published investigations in the foot and ankle literature involve consideration of the "therapeutic" model as described by the Oxford Center for Evidence-Based Medicine.
- Critical readers should appreciate the difference between a statistically significant difference and a clinically significant difference.

INTRODUCTION

One of the most important scientific lessons that a physician might learn is that while all studies have the ability to add to the ever-expanding body of medical knowledge, a study never has nor ever will *prove* anything. The concepts of "proof" and "truth" are primarily a matter of perspective and timing and not scientific fact. This admittedly philosophic maxim might be illustrated by asking readers to consider a seemingly simple question: Can you *prove* that the Sun is at the center of our solar system? On the surface, this might seem like a ridiculous query. All of us have lived in a period of time where this is an accepted, unquestioned fact. The scientific history of this question, however, might demonstrate an important lesson as it relates to foot and ankle science.

Department of Surgery, Temple University School of Podiatric Medicine, 148 North 8th Street, Philadelphia, PA 19107, USA
E-mail address: ajmeyr@gmail.com

Clin Podiatr Med Surg 41 (2024) 215–222
https://doi.org/10.1016/j.cpm.2023.07.003
0891-8422/24/© 2023 Elsevier Inc. All rights reserved.

One of the most accomplished and celebrated observational scientists of their time was the now nearly forgotten *Tycho Brahe* (1546–1601). A Danish astronomer, his measurements and recordings of celestial and planetary motions were so accurate that some are still in use today despite the fact that he died 7 years before the telescope was invented! After years and years of meticulous nightly data collection, he was able to derive a complicated description of the solar system in which the Earth sat as an immobile center, the stars were a fixed background, and the Sun and planets rotated about the Earth along complex differing orbits. Mathematically his model was astonishingly accurate and was praised accordingly. On the basis of his data set, again so advanced and accurate that it is still at least partially in use today, his description of the solar system with Earth as the center was accepted as "proof" and "truth" during his time and beyond.

In the years after this model became accepted scientific fact, an assistant at Brahe's laboratory by the name of *Johannes Kepler* (1571–1630) (a name that readers might be more familiar with) analyzed the same data set and derived the heliocentric model of the solar system which we would all recognize today. These 2 scientists used the same data set and derived similar mathematical accuracy with respect to their descriptions but arrived at 2 radically different conclusions. So which scientist was right and which was wrong? Is the Sun or the Earth at the center of our universe or solar system? The complicated answer is that they both were! Brahe was mathematically accurate and considered "right" at the time but "wrong" now, while Kepler was mathematically accurate but considered "wrong" at the time and "right" in contemporary history.

Although we still remember, teach, and celebrate the name Kepler today, it turns out that he also fell short of the concept of absolute truth. If Kepler was actually right, then none of us would have ever heard of Isaac Newton, who modified and refined Kepler's theory. And if Newton was actually right, then none of us would have ever heard of Albert Einstein, who modified and refined Newton's theory. And so on throughout the history of science. "Proof" is a matter of perspective and timing, and there is no doubt that we all possess a recency bias and publication bias that current knowledge is absolute "truth."

LEVELS OF CLINICAL EVIDENCE

This admittedly long-winded introduction has relevance with respect to contemporary interpretation of the clinical levels of evidence that serve as a pillar for critical analysis of the medical literature and evidence-based practice. Generally speaking, the profession of foot and ankle surgery uses a model for the levels of evidence similar to that used by the rest of medicine. **Table 1** shows a widely accepted description for the levels of clinical evidence in therapeutic studies. In other words, study methodologies that involve a specific patient intervention for a specific pathology. This likely represents an overwhelming majority of the published peer-reviewed studies in the podiatric literature.[1] The table is modified from, but consistent with, the Oxford Centre for Evidence-Based Medicine, the author guidelines of the Journal of Foot and Ankle Surgery, and the author's guidelines of the Journal of the American Podiatric Medical Association.[2–5]

With that said the author believes that there is an inaccurate perception currently imbued within the profession that relatively higher levels of evidence should be considered "right," "correct," and "good", while relatively lower levels of evidence are considered "wrong" and "bad." Just as Tycho Brahe and Johannes Kepler were simultaneously "right" and "wrong," contemporary investigators and critical readers should

Table 1	
Level of clinical evidence for interventional studies	
Level of Evidence	**Therapeutic/Interventional Studies**
1	High-quality randomized controlled trials; systematic reviews of homogenous Level 1 randomized controlled trials
2	Low-quality randomized controlled trials; prospective comparative studies; systematic review of Level 2 studies
3	Retrospective comparative studies; case–control studies; systematic reviews of Level 3 studies
4	Case reports and case series
5	Expert opinion

appreciate that the same holds true for the published literature. A Level 1 study is not "perfect," "good," "correct," or relatively "right" or "better" than a Level 4 study. Instead, it comes with a specific set of limitations inherent to all Level 1 methodologies. In a similar manner, a Level 4 study is not "bad," "wrong," or "worse" in comparison to a Level 1 study. Instead, it comes with its own specific set of limitations inherent to Level 4 methodologies. No study is perfect, and each and every study published in the medical literature has limitations. Therefore, the key to effective critical analysis of the medical literature is not to reject a study because of its limitations, but instead to actively identify these limitations and embrace how they will affect one's individual interpretation of the results.

In fact, one might argue that it is basic logic. If a reader rejects the results of *one* study because of the limitations, then they must therefore also reject the results of *all* studies as all studies have limitations. And conversely, if a reader can accept that one study might add to the body of knowledge, then they must also accept that all studies might add to the body of knowledge regardless of the level of evidence. In other words, Level 1 studies are not "right," whereas Level 4 studies are "wrong," but rather we might have a different level of confidence in the results of Level 1 studies in comparison to the results of Level 4 studies. This concept represents the intended overall theme of this edition of *Clinics in Podiatric Medicine and Surgery*. Readers are encouraged to reject a dualistic right or wrong approach to podiatric science and instead embrace a broader scientific view. Each of the authors for the following chapters has been challenged with bringing *Clinics* readers a practical and wide application of their specific material.

This theme, one might argue, is more in line with an "evidence-based approach." There is not always, and in fact rarely is, a single correct answer to a given clinical question. Instead, as physicians, we need to evaluate all available evidence and come to the best possible answer for a specific situation and with an individual patient. In a similar way, an article will rarely, if ever, provide a single answer to a specific clinical hypothesis. Instead, a good study will provide some evidence, but nearly always ask more questions than it will answer.

Types of Studies

The first thing to appreciate from **Table 1** is that it only speaks to therapeutic or interventional study methodologies. In fact, an expanded table is available which additionally describes the levels of evidence for different study methodologies including prognostic studies, diagnostic studies, and economic or decision analyses.[2,3] These methodologies are equally important certainly, but might not be as high yield as therapeutic studies for critical readers of podiatric literature. Therapeutic methodologies represent direct patient interventions fundamental to our profession such as the effects of surgical procedures, oral or intravenous medications, topicals, injections, and off-loading devices.

Levels of Evidence

This section will detail the specific differences in the levels of evidence for therapeutic interventions. As a practical example, the clinical concept of an "Achilles tendon rupture" will be used to detail how a single clinical situation might derive varying levels of evidence depending on the specific question that is asked by investigators.

LEVEL 5 EVIDENCE

Level 5 evidence is expert opinion. In other words, no original data are presented and no comparisons of unique data are performed. Examples of expert opinion include review articles, tips or quips or pearls, professional experiences, textbook chapters, professional lectures, and so forth. Using the example of an "Achilles tendon rupture," a Level 5 study might describe a new suturing technique for end-to-end repair of the ruptured tendon. The use of the new suturing technique is not clinically followed in any actual tendon ruptures, but the specific steps and potential advantages of the technique might be described.

In an evidence-based world, it might be relatively easy to dismiss Level 5 evidence as unscientific. However, most of what is learned in the practice of medicine comes from accrued experience and trial and error. The best and most well-received lectures at the American College of Foot and Ankle Surgeons Annual Scientific Conference, for example, is Level 5 evidence. A chapter from McGlamry's *Comprehensive Textbook of Foot and Ankle Surgery* (and indeed any article published in *Clinics in Podiatric Medicine and Surgery*) is Level 5 evidence. Although relatively low on the clinical level of the evidence grading system, these examples represent potentially substantial and perhaps the most common learning opportunities for most physicians in contemporary practice.

LEVEL 4 EVIDENCE

Level 4 evidence includes case reports and small case series. This category emphasizes that the primary differentiation between differing levels of evidence is based on what specific comparison is performed. In both case reports and case series, the only comparison is before and after a specific intervention. Perhaps surprisingly, it matters relatively little whether the intervention was performed on a single patient or on 500 patients. The comparison of pre- to post-intervention in a single cohort defines this level of evidence. The specific difference between a case report and a case series lies in the number of subjects investigated. Although the term "case report" might seem to imply a single patient, in practice, a case report involves up to approximately 20 patients presenting in a similar manner with respect to their diagnosis and/or intervention. Less than this approximate number is a case report, whereas more than that approximate number constitutes a case series.

Using the example of an "Achilles tendon rupture," perhaps the new suturing technique for end-to-end repair is used on a series of 25 patients. Outcome measures might include the amount of time it takes to return to a pre-injury level of activity, re-rupture rates, pain scores, functional outcome scores, Achilles tendon strength measurements, wound dehiscence rates, satisfaction rates, and so forth. Although the specific outcome measure is important with respect to what conclusions might be gleaned from the study, it is relatively inconsequential when considering the level of evidence. This methodology would be considered Level 4 evidence in that there is a single group of patients with a comparison of outcomes before and after the Achilles tendon repair.

The sixth (A New Paradigm in Foot and Ankle Outcomes?: Away from Radiographs and Towards Patient-centered Outcomes), twelfth (Unique Challenges in Diabetic Foot Science), and thirteenth (Special Considerations in Foot and Ankle Science: Translational Research, Dermatology, Gait Analysis, Cadavers and Databases) chapters of this *Clinics* edition provide a more in-depth look into the concept of outcome measures, whereas the seventh (Effective Case Reports and Small Case Series) and eighth (Retrospective Studies: Cohort and Case Series) chapters describe the critical analysis of and limitations inherent to common Level 4 methodologies.

LEVEL 3 EVIDENCE

Level 3 evidence methodologies invoke an advanced comparison and include retrospective comparative studies, case–control studies, and systematic reviews of Level 3 studies. This relatively advanced comparison is between 2 differing groups as opposed to before and after intervention in a single group. Data are most often collected in a retrospective manner for this type of methodology and comparison.

Using the example of an "Achilles tendon rupture," perhaps the postoperative outcomes of the 25 patients from the previous Level 4 investigation of the new suturing technique are compared with 25 patients who underwent an Achilles tendon repair with a more traditional open Krakow suture technique. Both groups are similar in that they underwent Achilles tendon repair and postoperative outcomes are evaluated in both groups, but the comparison is between 2 groups with a different surgical technique as opposed to within a single group.

Another common situation involving a Level 3 methodology would be to divide a single group in some way based on their outcome. For example, perhaps 10 of the 25 patients from the previous Level 4 investigation of the new suturing technique suffered a re-rupture, whereas 15 of the 25 patients went on to a successful outcome. If the 10 patients with a complication are compared with the 15 patients without a complication, then an advanced comparison is used, and the previous Level 4 methodology turns into a Level 3 methodology.

This highlights the importance of developing a specific clinical hypothesis or question before an investigation is initiated. From the same group of patients with an Achilles tendon rupture, a Level 3 methodology might be derived from a question, whereas a Level 4 or 5 methodology might be derived from another (similar) question. Chapter 3 (Incorporating Research into a Busy Clinical Practice: A Practical Approach) of this *Clinics* edition provides some insight into the development of hypotheses, and chapter 8 (Retrospective Studies: Cohort and Case Series) describes the critical analysis of and limitations inherent to common Level 3 methodologies. Chapter 10 (The Cookbook Approach to Evidence Synthesis in Surgical Research) describes the critical analysis of and limitations inherent to systematic reviews.

LEVEL 2 EVIDENCE

Level 2 evidence methodologies similarly use an advanced comparison between different groups but do so with a more external control and usually in a prospective manner. This includes low-quality randomized controlled trials, prospective comparative studies, and systematic reviews of Level 2 studies. So-called low-quality randomized controlled trials might involve a multitude of factors such as poor rates of follow-up, improper randomization, lack of subject or investigator blinding, and inconsistent results.[2,3]

Level 2 evidence methodologies most commonly involve data collection in a prospective manner and further help highlight the concept of methodological "quality." When data are collected in a retrospective manner, the investigators can only access outcomes that were already collected in the past. One obviously cannot go back in time and perform a specific pre-operative radiographic measurement, for example, if the radiographic projection was not originally performed before the surgical intervention. Retrospective investigations are beholden to the original documentation before an investigation was planned or considered. But when data are collected in a prospective manner, then investigators can decide ahead of time which outcomes they want to collect data on. This can then be standardized for any patient presenting with the specific studied pathology.

Using the example of an "Achilles tendon rupture," perhaps 2 surgeons in a single group perform Achilles tendon repair in differing ways. One surgeon uses the new suturing technique, whereas the other surgeon prefers the Krakow suturing technique. A prospective investigation might be initiated where functional outcomes and dynamic strength testing of the repaired Achilles tendon are performed every 2 postoperative weeks. Because the study methodology was designed before the performance of surgery, a protocol for standardized data collection might be established and followed. This allows for "better" data collection and analysis between the 2 groups, but this would still be considered a "low-quality" prospective trial as patients are not randomized to the 2 groups (instead, one surgeon performs all cases involving the first surgical technique and another surgeon performs all cases involving the second surgical technique) and the investigators are not blinded to the intervention (each surgeon is obviously aware of the intervention that they performed). This introduces the potential for inherent biases as discussed in chapter 9 (Prospective Surgical Cohort Analyses) of this *Clinics* edition.

LEVEL 1 EVIDENCE

Level 1 evidence methodologies are high-quality randomized controlled trials and systematic reviews of homogeneous Level 1 randomized controlled trials. Using the example of an "Achilles tendon rupture" for the final time, perhaps patients are randomized to receive either the new suturing technique or the traditional Krakow technique. Further, the patients are blinded and therefore unaware of which suturing technique was performed on their tendon. A varied group of surgeons perform both techniques depending on the randomization outcome but do not follow the patients postoperatively. Instead, another surgeon, blinded as to which suturing technique was performed, sees the patients throughout the postoperative protocol and collects all data. And even further, strict inclusion or exclusion selection criteria are used to ensure evenly matched groups with respect to age, gender, activity level, comorbidities and so forth, and greater than 80% of patients followed up through the entire postoperative study protocol, and statistically significant differences between groups in the primary outcome measure are observed. Chapter 9 (Prospective Surgical Cohort Analyses) of this *Clinics* edition describes the critical analysis of and limitations inherent to these types of prospective cohort analyses.

Limitations of the Levels of Evidence

Although critical readers might appropriately feel more confident in the data and comparisons derived from higher levels of clinical evidence, once again, this does not necessarily imply that it is "better" or has more clinical utility. In fact, as the methodological protocols of higher levels of clinical evidence exert more control on the study design, it might also mean that the data and results are less generalizable and less applicable. Consider an investigation on surgical reconstruction of Charcot neuroarthropathy as a representative illustration. If a Level 1 evidence or Level 2 evidence methodologic protocol is designed, then there is likely to be a stringent set of selection criteria. For example, not all patients with Charcot neuroarthropathy deformity are likely to be included based on this diagnosis, but instead, many might be excluded based on comorbidities. This might include patients with uncontrolled hyperglycemia defined as a hemoglobin A1c greater than 8%, or those with evidence of peripheral arterial disease and/or history of revascularization, or those with an elevated creatinine on hemodialysis. These exclusions are perfectly appropriate and "better" for the data but might not be representative of the typical patient who walks into an office with Charcot neuroarthropathy on a given Friday afternoon. More methodological control generally means less broad application in daily practice.

As another potentially relevant example, one hallmark of a "high-quality" randomized controlled trial has traditionally been the inclusion of comparison to a placebo. This again might lead to "better" data from an evidence-based medicine standpoint, but it has relatively little clinical application. In actual practice, physicians are effectively never in a situation where medical decision-making involves a decision between an intervention and a placebo. Instead, physicians are generally placed in situations where medical decision-making involves a decision between several similar interventions. In this way, a Level 2 prospective comparative study might have more usefulness than a Level 1 high-quality randomized control trial despite being at a lower level of clinical evidence. This developing concept is known as comparative effectiveness research. This acknowledges that placebo-controlled comparative trials are expensive and time-consuming, while at the same time being relatively inefficient and impractical.

Statistical Significance Versus Clinical Significance

The second chapter (Basic statistics, statistical design, and critical analysis of statistics for surgeons) of this *Clinics* edition provides an introduction to statistical concepts for the preceding clinical levels of evidence. By way of conclusion to this introductory chapter, another inaccurate perception currently imbued within the profession (at least in the opinion of the author) is a relative overreliance on the concept of statistical significance and the *P*-value. When considering contemporary evidence-based practices, there might be an erroneous assumed belief that studies that demonstrate a *P*-value less than or equal to .05 are considered "correct" and "good," while studies that do not demonstrate a statistically significant difference are considered "wrong" or "bad." Make no mistake that the performance of comparative statistics, and the generation and interpretation of *P*-values, are of vital importance in the critical interpretation of the medical literature. But at the same time, it is important to appreciate that the *P*-value is a matter of mathematics and not necessarily clinical application. A specific comparative study methodology is likely to generate a *P*-value, but it is up to the study investigators and critical readers to interpret the meaning and value of that number. Chapter 10 (The Cookbook Approach to Evidence Synthesis in Surgical Research) of this Clinics edition provides further description of this bias of *publication*.

As an example, a common clinical hypothesis and study methodology in the podiatric literature is to evaluate the effect of a specific osteotomy on the correction of the hallux valgus deformity.[6] An osteotomy that decreases the first intermetatarsal angle from 19° to 13° in a group of at least 20 patients is likely to generate a statistically significant difference. This is formulaic and primarily a consequence of math. But at the same time, most critical readers would agree that this is not a clinically significant difference. In other words, although the intermetatarsal angle has mathematically decreased, it remains within an abnormal range at 13°. It is unlikely that both surgeons and patients would be happy with this postoperative outcome despite the statistical significance!

Instead, statistical significance represents the first step in the interpretation of results. A statistically significant difference is one in which there is likely to be a mathematical difference between 2 groups of numbers. After, and *only after* this has been established, should study investigators and critical readers attempt to determine the clinical significance of this difference. Statistical significance does not imply clinical significance, and no mathematical formula can determine clinical significance. Readers are encouraged to keep this in mind while reading subsequent chapters of this *Clinics* edition.

DISCLOSURE

The author has nothing to disclose.

REFERENCES

1. Meyr AJ. A 5-year review of statistical methods presented in the Journal of Foot & Ankle Surgery. J Foot Ankle Surg 2010;49(5):471–4.
2. Hasenstein T, Greene T, Meyr AJ. A 5-year review of clinical outcome measures published in the Journal of the American podiatric medical association and the Journal of foot and ankle surgery. J Foot Ankle Surg 2017;56(3):519–21.
3. Centre for Evidence-Based Medicine. https://www.cebm.ox.ac.uk/. Accessed 6/3/2023.
4. Author information. The Journal of Foot & Ankle Surgery®. https://www.jfas.org/content/authorinfo Accessed 6/3/2023.
5. Author Center. Journal of the American Podiatric Medical Association. https://japmaonline.org/page/authorcenter. Accessed 6/2/2023.
6. Meyr AJ. Clinical importance versus statistical significance, and correcting the scientific literature. J Foot Ankle Surg 2016;55(5):903.

Basic Statistics, Statistical Design, and Critical Analysis of Statistics for Surgeons

Andrew J. Meyr, DPM[a],*, Daniel Jupiter, PhD[b,c]

KEYWORDS

- Biostatistics • Comparative analysis • Descriptive statistical
- Comparative statistical

KEY POINTS

- An introductory understanding of statistical principles is essential for both study design and critical analysis of the medical literature.
- Descriptive statistics are intrinsic to most study designs and describe the specific characteristics of a group.
- Comparative statistics provide an objective comparison between different groups.
- Although a multiplicity of statistical tests are available, most studies in the foot and ankle literature use a relatively small number of different descriptive and comparative tests.
- All foot and ankle surgeons can learn a baseline knowledge of statistics to use in the critical analysis of the medical literature.

INTRODUCTION

On a fundamental level, statistics is a set of tools used in medical decision-making no different than how a scalpel or a sagittal saw is used in the operating room. No foot and ankle surgeon is born with the inherent ability to use a scalpel or sagittal saw; it requires training and practice throughout medical school and residency to develop practical proficiency. Statistics are no different. No foot and ankle surgeon is born with the inherent ability to perform, understand, and critically interpret them. Instead, it requires training and practice throughout the course of a career in medicine to develop a working proficiency. Unfortunately, it has been our experience that most foot and ankle surgeons are relatively apprehensive about taking the first step with respect

[a] Department of Surgery, Temple University School of Podiatric Medicine, 148 North 8th Street, Philadelphia, PA 19107, USA; [b] Department of Biostatistics and Data Science, University of Texas Medical Branch, 301 University Boulevard, Galveston, TX 77555-1311, USA; [c] Department of Orthopaedic Surgery and Rehabilitation, University of Texas Medical Branch, 301 University Boulevard, Galveston, TX 77555-1311, USA
* Corresponding author.
E-mail address: ajmeyr@gmail.com

Clin Podiatr Med Surg 41 (2024) 223–232
https://doi.org/10.1016/j.cpm.2023.07.004
0891-8422/24/© 2023 Elsevier Inc. All rights reserved.

to this. In fact, it might almost feel like a frightening prospect to tackle this uncharted territory.

In order to, perhaps, alleviate some of these concerns, we would initially challenge foot and ankle surgeons to consider statistics in terms of a more familiar subject: the hallux valgus deformity. We know that approximately 200 surgeries have been described for correction of this common deformity, and that more procedures and refinements of existing techniques are developed on a near daily basis. Imagine for a moment that you are a first-year resident excited to start learning hallux valgus surgery. It would be of relatively little value for you to attempt to perform each of these 200 surgeries during the course of your training. You would experience a great deal of variety but would not develop proficiency or confidence in any individual procedure. However, from an opposing perspective, it might be just as unproductive for you to only experience a single hallux valgus procedure during your residency training. You would learn this one procedure exceedingly well but would not be able to treat a range of hallux valgus deformities in a variety of patients. One might argue that you would be better served to experience a small handful of hallux valgus procedures during residency, with those procedures being considered appropriate for a range of indications. For example, a couple each of distal procedures, shaft procedures, proximal procedures, arthrodeses, and so forth. Although you might not perform a single procedure 200 times, this more measured variety of experience would better prepare you to think and act like a surgeon in clinical practice, rather than to think like a technician.

We would argue that this is the way that foot and ankle surgeons should approach statistics. You do not need to develop an expert knowledge in 200 different statistical tests on the level of a trained statistician with a Master's degree or PhD. However, for the same reason, it would be of substantial benefit to know more than just one. Perhaps bringing this point home, a contemporary review of *The Journal of Foot and Ankle Surgery* found that 84% of original research articles published during a 5-year period used descriptive statistics, whereas 68% of articles used comparative statistics.[1] Although close to 50 different comparative statistical tests were used in the published work during this period, only 5 tests were frequently used (defined as occurring in >10% of articles). This is a fitting parallel to our hallux valgus illustration. It would be arguably low yield to develop expertise in the 50 different statistical tests but perhaps much higher yield to focus on and better understand the 5 that were most commonly used.

The above represents the intention of this brief statistical review. We aim to provide readers with a straightforward overview of the most common descriptive and comparative statistical tests that they are likely to encounter in the foot and ankle surgical literature. By no means will we attempt to turn readers into statisticians but instead we hope readers will avoid apprehension and embrace a more clear understanding of statistics when contributing to and critically interpreting the medical literature.

DESCRIPTIVE STATISTICS

As the name implies, descriptive statistics attempt to describe specific characteristics of a group. In the foot and ankle literature, this likely and most commonly refers to a patient population with a specific pathologic condition or undergoing a specific intervention. Some descriptive statistics are relatively self-evident and are often learned even before physicians enter their undergraduate education. These include descriptors such as the mean, standard deviation, range, median, mode, and so forth. As such, there might be an inherent tendency to rely excessively on these specific descriptors even in inappropriate situations. As a blunt example, it would be 100% mathematically accurate to say that the mean (or average) human being on planet Earth has one testicle and one ovary. Although absolutely mathematically accurate, it in fact effectively describes not a single human being on planet Earth! As another example, this is much like how every American family has on average 1.13 children. As your authors are parents ourselves, we can certainly avow not understanding what having 0.13 children feels like!

Data Distributions

An incredibly important concept to appreciate is that the *distribution* and *type* of a variable describing a group plays a key role in determining which descriptive statistics should be reported to describe it. This facilitates understanding, interpretation, and critical analysis. The *mean, standard deviation*, and *range* are vitally important descriptive statistics, in fact "work horses" in the medical literature but are only useful and appropriate in the description of *continuous variables with normally distributed populations*. These distributions are visually represented by the classic bell-shaped curve when graphically depicted. Fortunately, many distributions within the foot and ankle literature at least roughly meet this definition. **Fig. 1** depicts a histogram (bar graph demonstrating frequencies) of the talar declination angle (TDA) taken from a group of 250 feet from subjects without a history of foot/ankle surgery.[2] Most people would

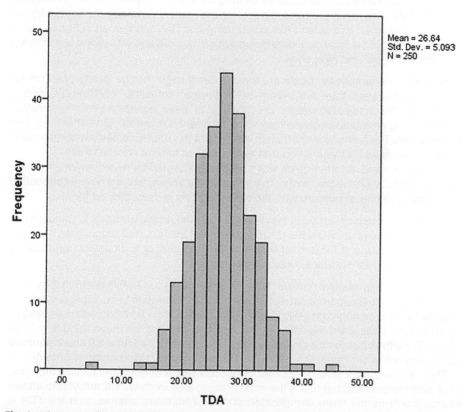

Fig. 1. Histogram (bar graph demonstrating frequencies) of the TDA taken from a group of 250 feet from subjects without a history of foot/ankle surgery.

look at this data distribution and agree that it looks at least roughly bell-shaped or normally distributed. There is a high point or apex at about 27°, and this falls off fairly equally on both sides of the apex.

Normally Distributed Populations

Interestingly, there is not a single accepted way or a single formula that determines whether a group of data points is normally distributed and would be appropriately described using the mean, standard deviation, and range. Moreover, although there is a relatively standard definition, if not entirely precise, for a normally distributed population (one in which 68% of the data is found within one standard deviation of the mean and 95% of the data is found within 2 standard deviations of the mean), one might argue that this is not a very practical definition in terms of making a determination of normalcy. Instead, there are multiple means that might be used to assess normality.[1]

- Graphically depict the data on a histogram as in the above example with the TDA. A reasonable subjective assessment might then be made of the distribution about whether it is normally distributed or not.
- Advanced statistics software can calculate the skewness and kurtosis of the data. A normally distributed population generally has a skewness and kurtosis, which are both between a range of −1 and 1.
- Statistical software might also be used to calculate a normal Q-Q plot to visualize the data. A normally distributed population is relatively close to the normal line on a Q-Q plot. An example of this again using our TDA is provided in **Fig. 2**.[2] Note how most of the individual data points fall on the solid line with only a few straying off at the low and high ends.

Although mathematically accurate, these 3 tests might not be overly practical for physicians because they are reliant on statistical software. Additionally, critical readers of the medical literature are unlikely to have access to this information when reading an article because they will not have the raw data. One effectively has to either take the author's word that an analysis of the data was performed to assess normality or make an assumption that the journal editor has ensured this.

With this in mind, another quick test might be performed by nearly anyone with access to a cellular phone calculator. This includes the investigators who are conducting the study, and critical readers who are reviewing one in its published form.

- If the standard deviation is less than 50% of the mean, and/or if 2 standard deviations above or below the mean fall inside of the reported range, then it is likely that the data is at least roughly normally distributed, or is close enough to be so considered for statistical reasoning purposes.

We can test this relatively simple "rule" by again using our TDA illustration. **Fig. 1** reports the mean to be approximately 27°, the standard deviation to be approximately 5°, and the range to be approximately 5° to 44°. This satisfies our first test because the standard deviation [standard deviation = 5] is less than 50% of the mean [27(0.5) = 13.5; 13.5 > 5]. Further, 2 standard deviations above the mean [27 + 2(5) = 37] and 2 standard deviations below the mean [27−5(2) = 17] fall within the reported range of 5° to 44°.

Thus, this relatively simple verification that can be performed with a calculator (and your authors promise that this is the most complicated math we will ask you to understand!) confirms the more complicated statistical software analysis that the TDA is probably a normally distributed distribution, and that it would be appropriate to describe it with the mean, standard deviation, and range.

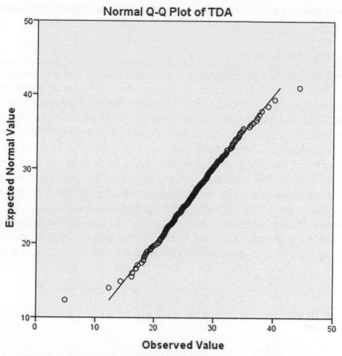

Fig. 2. A normal Q-Q plot might be generated by statistical software to visualize the normalcy of data. A normally distributed population will fall relatively close to the normal line on a Q-Q plot. Note how most of the individual data points fall on the solid line with only a few straying off at the low and high ends.

Confidence Intervals

Another commonly reported descriptive statistical, and one whose use has increased in frequency in contemporary descriptive statistics reporting, is the *confidence interval*. This tool offers precision in specifying the mean beyond that offered by the standard deviation and range alone. Moreover, from a practical standpoint for critical readers, it is difficult to conceptualize the presumed normal data distribution from the standard deviation and range (particularly if a histogram is not provided and/or data outliers are present). Confidence intervals consider the sample size, the mean, and standard deviation and effectively report both a range and a probability. So, at least intuitively if not completely accurately, for example, a 95% confidence interval indicates that there is a 95% chance that the measurement will fall within the interval. Any level of confidence might be calculated but it is most common to see a 95% confidence interval reported.

If we again use our example of the TDA from 250 feet, we observed a mean ± standard deviation (range) of approximately 27 ± 5 (5°–44°). Again, it might be difficult to conceptualize what the data distribution looks like based on this description. A confidence interval, however, describes the same data distribution and mean in a more "user friendly" manner. A standard formula calculates that the 95% confidence interval for this data to be approximately 27 ± 0.6. In other words, one can have 95% confidence that the mean TDA is between 26.4° and 27.6°. The 0.6 is specifically referred to as the *margin of error* and again considers the mean, standard deviation, and sample size.

One might also see this commonly reported with the following format: 27 (95% CI 26.4–27.6).

Nonnormal Data Distributions

Of course, not all data are normally distributed, and in fact, there is a huge variety of distributions that data might follow. Perhaps, the nonnormal distribution most commonly encountered by a podiatric physician is one with a *skewed right-sided* or *left-sided tail*. Take the calcaneal-cuboid angle (CCA) as an example (**Fig. 3**).[2] These are the same exact 250 feet from our previous example using the TDA but instead we now graphically depict the relationship between the calcaneus and the cuboid. Note how the graph looks roughly bell-shaped with an apex at approximately 10° but the data on the left side of the apex falls off sharply while the data on the right side of the apex falls off more gradually. Most people would evaluate this graph and say that there seems to be a "tail" of data to the right side of the graph.

The graph also reports a mean of approximately 13°, standard deviation of approximately 7°, and range of approximately 1° to 36°. This fails our test of normalcy as the standard deviation [= 7] is greater than 50% of the mean [13(0.5) = 6.5; 6.5 < 7].

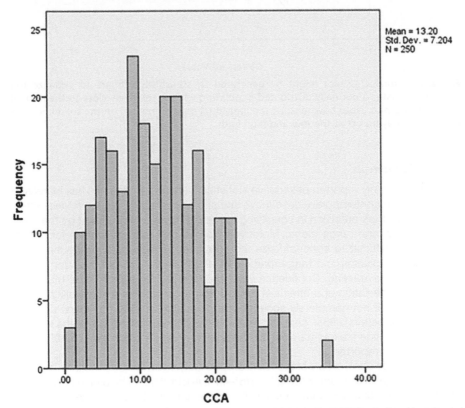

Fig. 3. Histogram of the CCA taken from a group of 250 feet from subjects without a history of foot/ankle surgery. Note how the graph looks roughly bell-shaped with an apex at approximately 10° but the data on the left side of the apex falls off sharply while the data on the right side of the apex falls off more gradually. Most people would evaluate this graph and say that there seems to be a "tail" of data to the right side of the graph.

Further, although 2 standard deviations above the mean $[13 + 7(2) = 27]$ falls within the range, 2 standard deviations below the mean $[13-7(2) = -1]$ does not.

Although this data might be "roughly" normally distributed, it would likely be more statistically accurate to consider this distribution to be nonnormal. In that case, it is less appropriate to describe the data in terms of the mean, standard deviation, and range but instead describe the data in terms of *median* and *interquartile range*. This determination of normalcy will also help determine which comparative statistical test is the most appropriate to use.

Frequency Counts and Percentages

A final common way to describe data is by means of a frequency count and percentage. Similar to the mean, this is also fairly common and likely familiar to anyone who has achieved a medical degree. Frequency counts are more appropriate when data is not *continuous* (like measuring degrees on a radiograph) but instead *categorical* (also referred to as *nominal*). This might be most common when the data variable is not necessarily measured but instead put into "buckets." Examples include male/female, diabetic/nondiabetic, satisfied/dissatisfied, and so forth.

The calculations involved here only require a basic calculator found on any cellular phone. Using our previous radiographic variable example, 116 of the 250 subjects were of male gender.[2] Therefore, it would be appropriate to report the frequency count as "116" and the percentage as "46.4% (116/250)".

Comparative Statistics

Speaking from personal experience, the aspect of statistics that seemed the most challenging to the corresponding author (AJM) when starting to learn these methods was the seemingly basic question of "Which comparative statistical tests should be used in which situations?" I read through and scoured dozens of different statistics textbooks in my residency's hospital library looking for an answer to this question, and unfortunately tended to end up more confused after each book! It was not until I came across the book, *Primer of Biostatistics*, by Stanton Glantz that my question was answered.[3] Surprisingly, no scouring of the book was even required. A chart (which I have modified and included below as **Table 1**) answering the question can be found on the inside cover.

With this personal admissions in mind, I am going to make a further statement that will surely make my respected biostatistician coauthor (DJ) cringe: in order to both perform and critically interpret the majority of the medical literature encountered by podiatric physicians, *comparative statistics are effectively a basic kitchen blender* (and cringe he did!). Given the ready availability of advanced and powerful statistical software, the derivation of and manual performance of specific comparative statistical tests is relatively inconsequential to the practicing foot and ankle surgeon. What is arguably more important is understanding how to appropriately arrange the data within the software (this is synonymous with adding the proper ingredients into the blender) and knowing which test to tell the software to run (this is synonymous with deciding which button on the blender to push: *puree* vs *liquefy*, for example). The software will then inevitably spit out a P-value similar to the way a blender mixes up a smoothie! However, add the ingredients in the wrong order or add the wrong ingredients… and the blender gives you something unpalatable.

I (AJM) could not begin to tell you the formulaic differences between the paired t-test and the Wilcoxon signed-rank test like Dr Jupiter could, for example, but I can tell you in which situations it is more appropriate to use each test. I think that is the real value in foot and ankle surgeons practically using **Table 1**. Basically, only 2 pieces of information

Table 1
Which comparative statistical tests are appropriate for which methodologies?

	Continuous Data	Ordinal Data	Categorical Data
Data description	Data that has equal, constant, and ordered intervals. This table assumes that interval data describes a normally distributed population	Data that has ordered intervals, but intervals that are not equal. Also includes continuous data with a nonnormal distribution	Data with arbitrary or nonarithmetic intervals
Before and after a single intervention in one group of the same individuals	Paired t-test	Wilcoxon signed-rank test	McNemar's test
Before and after multiple interventions in one group of the same individuals	Repeated measures of analysis of variance	Friedman statistic	Cochrane Q
Comparing 2 groups consisting of different individuals	Unpaired t-test	Mann-Whitney U (Wilcoxon rank-sum test)	Chi-square or Fisher Exact test
Comparing 3 or more groups consisting of different individuals	Analysis of variance	Kruskal-Wallis test	Chi-square or Fisher Exact test†
Association between 2 variables	Pearson correlation; Linear regression	Spearman rank correlation	Odds-ratio; Relative risk

are required in order to know "which button on the blender to push": (1) what kinds of numbers are being used? and (2) what is the study design of the comparison?

Kinds of Numbers: Continuous, Ordinal, and Categorical

We have actually set the stage for this discussion with our previous discussion of the normality of data distributions. *Continuous data* refers to variables on a scale with equal and constant intervals taken from a normally distributed population. This is perhaps the most common continuous data encountered in foot and ankle surgery and examples include age, radiographic angles, millimeters, blood glucose, and so forth. Again, it is important to appreciate that the scale is equal and constant. So it would be fair to say that a patient with an intermetatarsal angle of 18° has double that of another patient with an intermetatarsal angle of 9°, or that someone aged 20 years is half that of someone aged 40 years.

Ordinal data (or ranked data) is on a scale but a scale that is not equal or constant. Another important caveat is that this might also include seemingly continuous data but that is from a nonnormally distributed population. Many patient-reported and functional outcome measures, including the American Orthopaedic Foot and Ankle Society (AOFAS) scale and visual analog scale, are likely best considered as ordinal data. An illustration of ordinal data that I frequently use with my students is ranking your favorite sports teams. I (AJM) am a big fan of the Florida Gators football team from Gainesville and the Chelsea Football Club from London. If these teams win on a given weekend, I am typically in a pretty good mood. If either of these teams lose on a given weekend, then I am typically pretty cranky! I like both of these teams, and I like them both about equally. In addition, honestly, depending on the season, sometimes I am a bit more invested in the Gators while other times I am a bit more invested in Chelsea. Probably my third favorite sports team is the Philadelphia Eagles but it really is a distant third place. When the Eagles win or lose, it is more of a shoulder shrug and does not affect my mood. Although I can rank these 3 teams in a 1-2-3 order, the intervals between them are not equal or constant; 1 and 2 are very close together, whereas 3 is way down the list. A medical example is cancer grades or stages.

Categorical data is noncontinuous and without a rank. Therefore, male/female, diabetic/nondiabetic, pregnant/not pregnant, success/failure, complications/no complications, and so forth are all common examples of categorical data. The data is placed in to a figurative "bucket" instead of on a scale.

We have already indirectly discussed these kinds of numbers in our discussion of data distributions. Based on this, it would be fair to say that continuous data might be best described in terms of the mean, standard deviation, and range, whereas ordinal data might be best described in terms of the median and interquartile range, and categorical data might be best described in terms of a frequency count and percentage. We can now also use these differentiations in kind of numbers to determine which *column* of **Table 1** to work within when deciding on an appropriate comparative statistical test.

What Is the Study Design of the Comparison?

Determining the appropriate *row* on **Table 1** is based on the specific comparison performed within the study methodology. The table provides 5 potential comparisons: (1) before and after a single intervention in one group of the same individuals, (2) before and after multiple interventions in one group of the same individuals, (3) comparing 2 groups consisting of different individuals (ie, before or after an intervention), (4) comparing 3 or more groups consisting of different individuals (ie, before or after an intervention), and (5) association between 2 variables. These study methodologies are discussed in reference to the clinical levels of evidence in the first article of this *Clinics* edition (Meyr AJ. A study never proves anything. Contemporary interpretation of the levels of clinical evidence and statistical significance. Clin Pod Med Surg). Although admittedly not completely inclusive of all possible comparative methodologies, your authors have found that this describes the overwhelming majority of methodologies observed in the foot and ankle literature.

SUMMARY

Answering these 2 basic questions (what kinds of numbers are being used and what is the methodology of the comparison) allows one to determine the correct column and row from **Table 1** and to make a determination of an appropriate statistical test to perform in the given situation. Even if this has been described at a relatively entrance-level, we feel confident it can help young investigators determine which comparative tests might be most appropriately performed, as well as critical readers to evaluate if an appropriate test was performed in a published study. We would also respectfully recommend several sources for interested readers to expand on their statistical knowledge.[3–8]

DISCLOSURE

The authors have nothing to disclose.

REFERENCES

1. Meyr AJ. A 5-year review of statistical methods presented in the Journal of Foot and Ankle Surgery. J Foot Ankle Surg 2010;49(5):471–4.
2. Meyr AJ, Wagoner MR. Descriptive quantitative analysis of rearfoot alignment radiographic parameters. J Foot Ankle Surg 2015;54(5):860–71.
3. Glantz SA, editor. Primer of biostatistics. sixth edition. New York: McGraw-Hill Medical Publishing Division; 2005.
4. User's guide to the medical literature. In: Guyatt G, Rennie D, Meade MO, et al, editors. Essentials of evidence-based clinical practice. Second edition. New York: McGraw-Hill Medical; 2008.
5. Stengel D, Bhandari M, Hanson B, editors. Statistics and data management. A practical guide for orthopaedic surgeons. Switzerland: Thieme AO Publishing; 2009.
6. Riegelman RK, Hirsch RP, editors. Studying a study and testing a test. How to read the health science literature. Third Edition. Boston: Little, Brown and Company; 1996.
7. How to report statistics in medicine. In: Lang TA, Secic M, editors. Annotated guidelines for authors. Second edition. And reviewers. Second edition. Philadelphia: American College of Physicians; 2006.
8. Evidence-based medicine. In: Friedland DJ, Go AS, Davoren JB, et al, editors. A framework for clinical practice. New York: Lange Medical Books/McGraw-Hill; 1998.

Incorporating Research into a Busy Clinical Practice
A Practical Approach

Erin E. Klein, DPM, MS[a,b]

KEYWORDS

- Clinical research • Prospective studies • Evidence-based practice
- Protocol implementation

KEY POINTS

- To the well-trained mind who is critical of their results, research is the next logical step in validating a new or innovative treatment protocol(s).
- Planning is key to research protocols to being successful.
- Research workflows should be parallel to current patient care workflows.
- Writing complete and accurate notes that can be used by any member of the research team is crucial to retrospective reviews of prospectively collected data being useful.

INTRODUCTION

Research in active clinical practice is necessary and can be exceptionally valuable when studies are properly designed and executed. There is a considerable difference between the theoretically perfect research study and the real life that occurs in the busy clinic. When one is in clinic, patients are probably having "bad" days when they are in pain, distressed, depressed, and/or possibly anxious over their medical condition.[1] This creates challenges in data collection that are conquerable with proper planning. The key to collecting data in a busy clinical practice is to understand that data will not always be ideal but less than perfect data is both valuable and useable in high-level research projects. The goal of this article is to provide a framework for efficient day-to-day research data collection and subsequent publication.

How do I Determine what to Study? Start with Your Everyday

The best ideas for research studies come from the day-to-day lives of busy clinicians. There are problems that will develop in the lives of patients that may not have a clear

a Weil Foot & Ankle Institute, 1660 Feehanville Road, Mount Prospect, IL 60056, USA; b Dr William M Scholl College of Podiatric Medicine at Rosalind Franklin University of Medicine and Science, North Chicago, IL, USA
E-mail address: eek@weil4feet.com
Twitter: @weil4feet (E.E.K.)

Clin Podiatr Med Surg 41 (2024) 233–238
https://doi.org/10.1016/j.cpm.2023.10.001
0891-8422/24/© 2023 Elsevier Inc. All rights reserved.

treatment or solution based on the existing evidence-based literature. The clinician may be observing things that he/she/they cannot find in the literature. Research starts here—with the problems and the pathology that is present every day.

Innovative solutions are a part of the podiatric practice; however, many of these innovations lack substantive research because the busy clinician/surgeon may not have a proper framework for systematic evaluation of the results of care. This article focuses on ways to create clinic protocols that allow clinical research to be conducted in a way that is conducive to patient care in a busy, non–hospital-based clinic.

PLANNING: PRIOR PLANNING PREVENTS POOR PERFORMANCE

Prior planning prevents poor performance. Planning is the key to successful completion of research studies.

What are the requirements for research oversight in your area?

Research may require the approval of an Institutional Review Board (IRB). Many large hospital systems and university type settings will have an internal IRB. In more rural areas, this may not be the case and you may need to find an IRB (virtual or online) to review your study before implementation. Each IRB has processes and procedures that are specific to that organization. These concepts are reviewed in Ansert, and colleagues, later in this edition of *Clinics*.[2]

Research protocols need to be reviewed by the IRB. Some studies will require a full board review, whereas others will be determined to be "exempt" from a full board review. Even if your study is deemed to be "exempt" from review, it is still important to submit that application so that the IRB is aware of what you are doing.

As part of the IRB process, there is generally a requirement for Human Subjects training. It is important to contact your IRB to determine their requirements. If your IRB is based at a university or hospital system, they may have internal training that is required. If your IRB is virtual or online, they may require specific online training. Generally, this type of training must be updated annually.

What is your objective?

One must start with an objective. Initially, this does not have to be very specific. Starting with a slightly broader objective might have advantages as a broader range of data will be collected. Once you have data, you can determine what you need to use and future directions. It is better to have data that you do not need rather than to need data that you do not have.

It is also important to determine if you are collecting data on one pathology or if you are trying to create a database/repository of prospectively collected data for retrospective review. These 2 categories of investigations have different publication requirements but similar implementation processes.

What is your patient population?

Quality research requires statistics. Demonstrating statistically significant differences in research studies typically requires a specific number of patients. It is prudent and critical that studies have the correct number of patients/subjects to support the conclusion(s) of the study. Obtaining this "critical mass" of patients/subjects starts before data collection by identifying if you/your institution have the necessary number of patients. For example, if your research team seeks to conduct a study on sequela of total ankle replacements but only performs 10 total ankle replacements a year, this may not be the proper topic of study. However, if your research team seeks to identify how many patients with plantar fasciitis progress to surgical management of this condition and plantar fasciitis is the most common pathologic condition that is seen in the office, then a study would be easier to conduct and will likely have the necessary numbers to observe statistically significant outcomes.

Most electronic medical record (EMR)/electronic health record (EHR) software has reporting features that allow creation of reports based on international classificaiton of diseases, 10th edition (ICD-10) and/or current procedural terminology (CPT) codes. These can be exceptionally helpful in gauging if desired studies are feasible. This is a very efficient and effective way to identify a patient population; however, weaknesses exist. First, ICD-10 codes must be accurate. If you were looking to study plantar fibromas, the ICD-10 code M72.2 would be accurate. However, this code is also used for plantar fasciitis. A member of the study team would need to sort through notes to determine which patients belonged to which group. Similarly, there are times where different procedures are coded with the same CPT code (ie, Austin bunionectomies and reverdin bunionectomies). This would require reviewing operative reports to assure the correct procedure is studied. The use of technology for this purpose is exceptionally helpful; however, all reports must be verified if the authors are to assure accuracy of the data.

What is your support structure?

Research should be a group project. Physicians need to perform the duties of the physician. Research projects require additional support. In the team approach, each member of the team is responsible for specific tasks. This leads to a more robust data collection that is not overly stressful on any one member of the team. The number of staff needed will vary based on the exact nature of the research study.

Each research team should contain a person who understands how to structure EMR/EHR data so that the data that are entered can be easily extracted. Exactly how this is done is specific to the EMR/EHR. It has been the author's experience that understanding the capabilities of your technology is important to being able to do certain portions of research studies more efficiently.

Each research team should have frequent contact with a statistician. This person's role on the team is to review the study protocol before it is implemented to assure that the variables measured are clear, specific, and able to be analyzed. Further, this person should assist with assuring that the study outcomes support the conclusions.

Once the team has been identified, implementation of a clinical workflow to support your study needs can begin.

HOW TO EFFECTIVELY COLLECT DATA DURING PATIENT CARE VISITS

This topic can be very overwhelming but it does not have to be. The following part of this article is aimed to break each part of the patient visit down to where and how you can collect data without causing major disruption in clinic flow.

Establish a research workflow that is complementary and parallel to current patient care workflows. Clinic can be busy and chaotic. Establishing complimentary workflows allow more work to be done in the same amount of time creating efficiency. Spreading the responsibilities throughout the team should not overburden or overwhelm any individual team member.

Each person(s) discussed in the following paragraphs has specific responsibilities. Each person(s) should have a mechanism to hold each other accountable for their research responsibilities.

Many physicians have patient care protocols and workflows to help with clinic efficiency. If these types of protocols are not currently in place, it might be prudent to start with patient care protocols before trying to implement research protocols.

Prior to clinic, all patients should be screened for ongoing research studies. Screening is typically performed by a medical assistant or research coordinator in the day or week before clinic. This process allows anyone who may be eligible to participate in a study to be contacted before they arrive in clinic. This works best with patients who are already established with the physician/practice. Once the patient agrees to review study materials to see if they are interested, the medical assistant or coordinator can email the patient the informed consent and any informational material on the study. This allows patients time to process the information and form questions at their own pace. The hope is that this decreases the stress and anxiety of medical care and allows more information to be exchanged at the patient's clinic visit.

Data collection can begin with *new patient paperwork and the intake process*. Demographics (age, biological sex, zip code of residence, and so forth) and health history are frequently reported on paper or a kiosk. If you are looking at specific variables, make those variables mandatory and do not allow the patient to proceed without entering those variables. Health history (past medical history, past surgical history, allergies, medications, social history, and so forth) should be specific as possible, and this may require a member of the health-care team to review, condense, and clarify any EMR/EHR-based problem lists. Vital signs—including height and weight—should be accurately measured, not estimated, and then recorded in the EMR/EHR. Patient-reported outcome measures (ie, Foot and ankle outcome score,[3,4] SF-12,[4] SF-36,[4] and so forth) can be included in your new patient paperwork. This will allow for a baseline measurement for all patients and serve as a "prescreening" for current research studies.

The *morning huddle* is how many clinics start a day. This allows the clinical staff to determine the needs of each patient during the day. Add identification of research patients and the specific needs of these research patients into this huddle. This way, all team members are aware and empowered to assist with data collection. Clear direction and responsibilities for each patient visit that day should be established at the morning huddle. This will allow all team members to have clarity, direction, and focus during patient care.

Patients check in at a *front desk or a reception area*, and this is typically followed by some amount of waiting. This is a great time to collect data. If you are using surveys or patient-reported outcome measures, this is a time where patients are a captive audience and data can be collected. The authors have found that it is easiest to collect data when the patient is physically present in the office.

It is research team/institution dependent if data are collected electronically on an iPad or similar device versus being collected on paper. Electronic collection frequently means that the data from the iPad or similar device is put into a spreadsheet (or something similar) in an automated fashion. Comparatively, data collected on paper requires legible handwriting and that the answers to the survey questions be manually entered by a member of the research team into a spreadsheet. There is the additional consideration of where to physically store these surveys after they are collected that is IRB and Health Insurance Portability and Accountability Act (HIPAA) compliant.

After the lobby/reception area, patients are greeted by a *medical assistant or a nurse*. This person is a member of the research team even if they do not know it. The nurse or medical assistant is responsible for vitals, data entry into the patient's chart (ie, visual analog pain scale or other pain scale score, pathology-specific measures of health, health history, and so forth), taking radiographs, and uploading imaging studies. It is important that medical assistants and nurses know what data are required for your study (ie, visual analog pain scale scores, survey instruments, and pathology-specific questions) so that this individual can get the proper information into the patient's chart (or any other research program or spreadsheet). The medical assistant or nurse should be aware of what is occurring that day for both patient care *and* research.

The patient should then be seeing their *physician/surgeon*. It is critical that this provider is invested in the research component of practice. This requires knowledge of which patients are "research patients" and what is required for each of these patients. During the patient visit, the physician/surgeon should be conducting a patient care visit while asking questions critical and appropriate to research.

Following patient visits, physicians write notes. Research studies will only work if physician notes are accurate and personalized to that patient encounter. Notes must contain the correct information for that visit and the research study. Finally, notes must be written in a way that is understandable. EMR/EHRs can make this process easier; however, it is important that notes are personalized to the patient. The use of templates or prepopulated notes can hinder research if every note is the same because it does not allow for patients to deviate from the standardized or protocoled course.

EMRs/EHRs may have the capability to extract information from patient notes. Many software companies have a way of writing notes that structures information in a way that the reporting part of the software should be able to extract the required information without a person reading notes, per se. As noted above, the ICD-10 and CPT coding can be used to identify patient populations. It is important that this data be as accurate as possible so that this process can be efficient and accurate.

Before the patient leaves the office, the medical assistant or clerical staff should ensure that all necessary paperwork and survey instruments are collected and labeled appropriately. Checklists can be very helpful for this task. Finding that one missing piece of information is much harder after the patient has left the office.

DATA ENTRY

As noted above, data can be collected at multiple points during the patient encounter. There needs to be a plan for data entry. The study statistician should be intimately involved in the process of creating the spreadsheets that will be used for data analysis. There are full books devoted to this topic, so a thorough discussion is beyond the scope of this article.

PUBLICATION

Writing is critical to communicating research findings. If a team is committed to creating questions, developing research projects, and collecting data, results should be communicated to the rest of the scientific community. Without this part of the process, patient care and science cannot grow.[5]

Although a full discussion of the publication process is beyond the scope of this article, there is one component of the publication that should be addressed early in the research study process—authorship. Each team/institution likely has a slightly different criterion for authorship. In many places, authorship can be a significant source of stress, particularly for younger researchers/physicians.[6]

PEARLS OF WISDOM

Research is a labor of the love of advancing science. To the well-trained mind who is critical of their results, research is the next logical step in validating a new or innovative treatment protocol. Research can be overwhelming at times—particularly when clinic days get busy or when life outside of work demands attention. We have found that patients are willing to participate in research, even if this means a slightly longer clinic visit, when they have a rapport with the physician and the clinical staff.

Life happens. Challenge yourself and your team to set up protocols that are based on solid patient care. This will assure that you are providing amazing patient care on days when research is furthest from your mind. Relying on technology to assist you is key because this can decrease your overall workload. When pursued with purpose, the outcome will be worth the entire journey.

CLINICS CARE POINTS

- Clinical research should be a team effort. Selecting team members with diverse backgrounds and expertise will allow the creation of a team where all members can contribute.
- Planning and discipline are the keys to successful completion of research studies.

DISCLOSURE

The author has nothing to disclose.

REFERENCES

1. Holt M, Swalwell CL, Silveira GH, et al. Pain catastrophizing, body mass index and depressive symptoms are associated with pain severity in a tertiary referral orthopaedic foot/ankle patients. J Foot Ankle Res 2022;15(1):32.
2. Ansert F, Crisologo P, Cates N, et al. Navigating institutional review boards. Clin Podiatr Med Surg 2023;41(2).
3. Joshi A, Collazo C, Laidley Z, et al. Validation of the foot and ankle outcome score for use in infracalcaneal heel pain. J Foot Ankle Surg 2023;62(3):501–4.
4. Safavi PS, Janney C, Jupiter D, et al. A systematic review of the outcome evaluation tools used in the foot and ankle. Foot Ankle Spec 2019;12(5):461–70.
5. Asnake M. The importance of scientific publication in the development of public health. Cien Saude Colet 2015;20(7):1972–3.
6. Norman MK, Proulx CN, Rubio DM, et al. Reducing tensions and expediting manuscript submission via an authorship agreement for early-career researchers: a pilot study. Account Res 2023;30(7):379–92.

Navigating Institutional Review Boards

Elizabeth Ansert, MA, DPM, MBA, AACFAS[a],*,
Nicole K. Cates, DPM, AACFAS[b], Andrew Crisologo, DPM, AACFAS[c],
Paul J. Kim, MS, DPM[c]

KEYWORDS

- Medical publications • Podiatric research • Research submission
- Human subject protections

KEY POINTS

- Institutional review boards have a common goal of protecting human subjects from physical or psychological harm during any research endeavor.
- Institutional review boards were created based on a history of poor research ethics and harm caused to research subjects.
- Institutional review boards can be local or central, both with advantages and disadvantages.
- Institutional review boards require specific documentation and materials for approval.
- Institutional review boards can allow for exemption, expedited reviews, or full reviews based on the participant's risk and research protocol.

INTRODUCTION
Background and Definitions

Research on human subjects has been historically plagued with perverse initiatives.. These events have occurred when investigators fail to recognize or protect human rights (**Fig. 1**). The Nuremberg trials resulted from the atrocities of World War II when German doctors performed detrimental experiments on prisoners. The Nuremberg Code stemmed from the USA vs Brandt trial specifically,[1] which created a 10-point ethical code for human research subjects.

[a] Department of Plastic Surgery, University of Texas Southwestern Diabetic and Limb Salvage, University of Texas Southwestern Medical Center, 5323 Harry Hines Boulevard, Dallas, TX 75219, USA; [b] Hand & Microsurgery Medical Group, 2299 Post Street, Suite 103, San Francisco, CA 94115, USA; [c] Department of Plastic Surgery, University of Texas Southwestern Medical Center, 1801 Inwood Road, Dallas, TX 75390, USA
* Corresponding author.
E-mail address: Eaansert@gmail.com

Clin Podiatr Med Surg 41 (2024) 239–246
https://doi.org/10.1016/j.cpm.2023.06.011
0891-8422/24/© 2023 Elsevier Inc. All rights reserved.

podiatric.theclinics.com

The History of Human Subject Protections

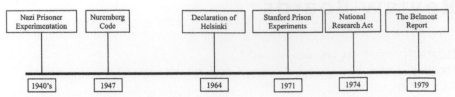

Fig. 1. A brief timeline of some important human subject protection events in recent history.

These 10 points included the following:

1. Voluntary consent
2. Yield meaningful results
3. Be based on animal studies or understanding of the disease
4. Avoid unnecessary suffering
5. A belief that death or disabling injury will occur
6. Risk should not exceed humanitarian importance
7. Preparations to protect the subjects should be done
8. Should be conducted by qualified persons
9. Voluntary termination of research by the subject
10. Researchers should terminate the experiment if a subject is being harmed

Despite the Nuremberg Code, several studies were performed following its enactment that demonstrated poor ethical decisions. In the United States, the Willowbrook study, the Tuskegee Syphilis study, and the Fernald States School trials are all examples of what is possible when research ethics are unchecked. In 1964, a meeting was held in Helsinki, Finland by the World Medical Association. A set of ethical principles was developed, and 10 specific topics were addressed, which included risks and benefits, vulnerable subjects, scientific requirements and protocols, ethics committees, confidentiality, informed consent, placebos, posttrial provisions, publication and dissemination of results, and unproven interventions in clinical practice. These principles became one of the cornerstones for ethical research as we know it today.

In 1971, a study took place that would become one of the most notorious examples of unethical investigations in recent history, despite the principles in place. Zimbardo conducted the Stanford prison experiment.[2] Participants would sustain substantial trauma from just 6 days of a simulated prison setup. Consequently, a growing public concern for the unethical treatment of research subjects developed. As a result, in 1974, the National Research Act was created by the National Commission for the Protection of Human Subjects of Biomedical and Behavioral Research. From this, the National Commission created the Belmont Report in 1979, which outlined basic ethical principles for human subjects' protection in biomedical and behavioral research.[3] There were 3 key principles: respect of persons, beneficence, and justice.

The Respect-for-Persons principle describes people as autonomous beings who can make their own decisions. This principle also notes that certain populations need additional safeguarding, as they do not have true autonomy. Patients with physical or mental illnesses, children, and prisoners are just *some* examples of research participants who need additional protection. These protections are extended until the participant becomes capable of self-determination. The second principle is beneficence. Simply, the benefits of the subject participating in the experiment should be maximized, whereas the risks should be minimized. The final principle is justice. The considerations of the participants should always come before the objective of the experiment. It also refers to the fair distribution of risks and benefits for participants, and no undue risks should be imposed.

The Belmont Principles, along with the Declaration of Helsinki, became the foundation of today's ethical research regulations. With the distribution and understanding of these principles, institutional review boards (IRBs) were formed to ensure that qualified persons reviewed a research study and verified its ethical merit before its induction. Traditionally, IRBs are formed within a specific institution. Central or independent IRBs have also developed to allow for practitioners without ties to an institution to conduct ethical research.

An IRB is made up of at least 5 members with varying backgrounds. All members assess a study's scientific method and ethical considerations. IRBs are required to have at least one member who has a scientific or physician background, one member who does not have a scientific background, and one who represents the community outside of the institution. The IRB is led by one chair. Depending on the institution, a vice-chair may also be present.

LOCAL INSTITUTIONAL REVIEW BOARDS

Often as rising investigators, one's first experience is with a local IRB through a hospital or academic institution. Local IRBs understand the nuanced complexities of its community because of specific ties and knowledge; this allows board members to have a deep understanding of the vulnerable populations, specific cultures, relevancies, and general ethical standards within that area. Local IRBs reflect the opinions and culture of the community from which the subjects are recruited, and this enables IRB members to evaluate the feasibility, strengths, and weaknesses of proposed research projects.[4]

In addition, local IRB members can be more accessible to ask questions, defend aspects of the study, and be a direct resource to the investigator for things such as supplies and recruitment. A local IRB will have a better understanding of the reputations and relationships of various people in the community, which could help guide the investigators to more successful outcomes. Local institutions see both the benefit of building a relationship with the community by establishing patient care and trust as well as the prestige and possible financial rewards of conducting ethically and methodologically sound research. Performing research may be welcomed in the community, as it brings resources, jobs, and clinical care to the area. It can also help to establish a practitioner within the area and possibly align them with members of the community if the research is performed ethically and correctly. Ultimately, local IRBs will place the protection and interest of the community and academic institution above all else.

However, local IRBs do have their limitations. Because local IRBs depend so much on their knowledge of the community, it can be difficult for a new researcher to be seen outside of the novice lens. In addition, a researcher may have a different way of practicing that is novel to the community. If a practitioner's reputation within the community is questioned, it could be difficult for the IRB to look past this and examine the research method independently. Although the IRB is ultimately trying to protect the subjects and community, having a predetermined opinion of a researcher could hinder or halt any forward progress in a project.

One other major consideration with local IRBs is that the reviews can often be slow and inconsistent. It is important to remember that very few, if any, members of the review board know the specifics of podiatric medicine. The members of the IRB may not be within the surgical or even medical specialty. Because of this, procedures and methods that may seem obvious to a podiatric specialist may be completely foreign to a member (or members) of the local IRB. One example comes from the authors' experiences. An IRB was submitted for a prospective study. After approximately 3 months of deliberation, the IRB returned a decision needing several points of clarification. One of the major revisions requested was to explain what a #15 surgical scalpel and surgical suture scissors were. The IRB wanted the make, model, company description, and patent of instruments described in the methodology. This example demonstrates that although the IRBs at a local level can have many advantages, there can also be some tedious tasks associated with the experience.

CENTRAL INSTITUTIONAL REVIEW BOARDS

Historically, researchers were required to obtain IRB approval from the institution at which they were conducting their research. However, some investigators are not associated with a particular institution. For those who do not have access to a local IRB, central IRBs have begun to fulfill this need. For example, a practitioner who works in a private office typically will have limited access to a local IRB. If someone wanted to study the effects of extracorporeal shockwave therapy on tendonitis, an IRB review would be required. A central IRB allows researchers in this circumstance to produce ethical research regardless of institutional ties; this broadens the opportunities for medical research to all practitioner types.

A central IRB may also be able to have more specialized reviewers or call on experts in a particular field. Experts in a particular specialty may allow for a keener review of the project while also understanding the nuances of the field, and this may help the other members of the IRB understand the field's standards and facilitate the board's understanding of the project.

Central IRBs do not come without their own inherent limitations and considerations. Most require a fee for the processing and review of the proposal. Critics have argued that this allows investigators to "shop around" or "buy" the answer that they want, ultimately questioning the integrity and merit of the review and approval. In addition, a central IRB does not replace a local IRB if a practitioner is associated with an institution. The local IRB may accept the central IRB approval, grant its own approval, reject it, or require revisions.

GETTING AND MAINTAINING INSTITUTIONAL REVIEW BOARDS
Review Types

All human subject study submissions must go through an initial review before the beginning of any data collection. There are various reviews that can be applied to different

Table 1			
Overview of institutional review board review types			
Review Type	Risk Level	Number of Reviewers	Example
Exempt	Minimal	One to a few	Anonymous surveys
Expedited	Minimal with sensitive information	Full	Retrospective chart review
Full	More than minimal risk	Full	Prospective drug study

types of research, depending on the potential risk to the participants (**Table 1**). On some IRBs, the chair of the board or a few members may briefly review the proposal to determine if an exemption, expedited review, or full review is warranted. Other IRBs may allow for administrative personnel to make this initial determination.

Some studies can be exempt from IRB review if they involve *minimal* risk to the participants. The types of studies are outlined in Title 45, Part 46 of the Code of Federal Regulations.[5] The Code of Federal Regulations defines minimal risk as "the probability and magnitude of harm or discomfort anticipated in the research are not greater in and of themselves than those ordinarily encountered in daily life or during the performance of routine physical or psychological examinations or tests."[5] The information must be completely anonymous, and any information obtained through the research would not harm the subject if that information was disclosed outside of research settings.

Expedited reviews typically involve no more than minimal risk to the participants but do not exhibit the criteria for an exemption. These studies can include retrospective or prospective chart reviews, surveys or observational studies that include sensitive information, and biospecimens whose patient information is not public.

The most extensive review is referred to as a full study. A full review is needed when a study involves more than minimal risk to the subjects or involves a protected population, such as those who cannot give informed consent. This review is often needed with prospective studies, especially if an intervention is invasive.

Materials for Initial Reviews

Every IRB will have its own requirements for proposals. One of the first steps in obtaining IRB approval is to learn the specific requirements needed for a particular IRB. However, there are documents that can be considered standard for most proposals. First, most IRBs require a submission form, protocol, human subject training certification, curriculum vitae, a professional license for the principal investigator, and a copy of the subject consent form. If a drug or device is being tested or used, the IRB may require the drug or product information, brochures, or other supplemental material. Some IRBs may also require a conflict-of-interest statement or financial disclosure form to be included for the initial review.

The submission form and protocol form can often be the same document for local IRBs. For central review boards, these forms may be separated into 2 distinct documents. Information that is often needed in protocols includes the following:

- Name and educational backgrounds of all investigators
- The purpose or objective of the study
- Design of the study
- Location of study
- Informed consent
- How and what information will be obtained
- How that information will be deidentified and stored/protected
- Statistical analysis plan
- Materials used
- The benefits and risks to the participants

The IRB may also require a brief literature review, justification for the study, and how it would add to the current literature. **Box 1** gives a brief overview of a previous IRB protocol submission form from an investigator's local institution. Ultimately, the materials required for the initial review can be dependent on the IRB and the specifics of the study. It is best to contact the review board directly in most cases to ask for a list of what is needed to help expedite the process. Review boards may have this

---

Box 1
A protocol template example from previous institutional review board submissions

1. Protocol Title:
2. Investigator(s):
3. Version Date:
4. Objectives:
5. Background:
6. Setting of the Research:
7. Resources Available to Conduct this Research:
8. Study Design:
   a. *Recruitment Methods*
   b. *Inclusion and Exclusion Criteria*
   c. *Study Endpoints*
   d. *Procedures Involved in the Research*
   e. *Data Management*
   f. *Provision to Monitor the data for the Safety of Subjects*
   g. *Withdrawal of Subjects*
9. Statistical Plan
   a. *Sample Size Determination*
   b. *Statistical Methods*
10. Risks to Subjects
11. Potential Benefits of Subjects
12. Provisions to Protect the Privacy Interests of Subjects
13. Provisions to Maintain the Confidentiality of DATA
14. Medical Care and Compensation for Injury
15. Cost to Subjects
16. Consent Process
17. Vulnerable Populations
18. Sharing of Results with Subjects
19. References
20. Attachments

---

information available online, especially if they are a central IRB. Most institutions will also have a central web-based portal where documents are submitted.

Once an initial review has been completed and all materials are submitted, the IRB will determine what type of review is warranted and if any additional materials are needed. If the IRB approves the protocol, an official approval letter is sent to the researchers with a specific approval number. However, the IRB may require that the proposal be revised or that researchers provide additional information or clarification. On rare occasions the principal investigator may be asked to be present at an IRB meeting to address any questions directly. In the authors' experiences, materials specific to instruments used, revisions to protecting patient information or location, and questions regarding the justification of the study have been a few areas that required clarification or expansion. When this happens, the IRB will ask for a document that addresses each concern raised by the IRB, which are to be responded to directly. If additional materials are required, these are submitted in separate, labeled documents and referenced within the query response. The IRB can then continue to inquire more information, approve the revision, or reject the project.

Maintaining Approval and Close-Out

Once approval from the IRB is received, it is expected that the protocols are being followed. If there is a deviation in protocol, a breach of confidentiality, a discovered conflict of interest, adverse event, or any changes that are wished to be made, the IRB is required to be formally informed in a timely fashion. Based on the nature of the request or deviation, appropriate action is determined by the board. The IRB must also be renewed, usually on a yearly basis. This process can be specific to the institution, but typically the initial application and progress of the study is submitted.

An example an investigator has with protocol modification is adding an investigator to an existing study. A formal proposal was made to a local IRB to add the investigator to the protocol. The IRB required the investigator's human subject training certification, professional license, curriculum vitae, and what this investigator would contribute to the project. The investigator was not allowed to participate in the research until they were approved to be added to the project. Once approved, a formal letter from the IRB chair was issued, and the new investigator was allowed to participate in the study.

Adverse events are also considered when maintaining approval and/or closing out a study. The Office for Human Research Protections defines an adverse event as "any untoward or unfavorable medical occurrence in a human subject, including any abnormal sign, symptom, or disease, temporally associated with the subject's participation in the research, whether or not considered related to the subject's participation in the research."[6] Often, adverse events are required to be reported within 2 weeks to an IRB. However, some regulations require reporting sooner. Serious adverse events are often considered life-threatening, requiring medical treatment, or causing significant disability. These events are usually required to be reported in 1 week. Deaths are typically required to be reported in 24 hours. Maintaining approval and closing studies will require an adverse event report.

When a research project is concluded, an IRB closeout is often required; this can be due to completion of an experiment, termination of a project before its completion, or a study that was not and will not be initiated. A study is closed when access to and use of identifiable data is completed. Data can still be analyzed, and articles can be written after the IRB is closed. Many institutions require a form or closeout report. This report can include institution-specific questionnaires, principal investigator assurances, supporting documentation, outcomes of the study, and any other required material—this can vary by institution or IRB approval granting body, so it is important to review what requirements a specific IRB has during this stage of the IRB.

CLINICS CARE POINTS AND PEARLS

- IRBs are filled with both researchers and nonresearchers who are often not familiar with the podiatric field. It is important to start the IRB process early, ask what materials will be needed in advance, and be patient throughout the process.

- Local IRBs are more in touch with local community nuances and likely better able to serve their community.

- Central review boards are an alternative for practitioners not associated with an institution seeking to perform ethical studies.

- IRB submissions have specific guidelines to follow. Obtain a template from the board you are seeking approval from to follow their outlines for the most straight forward process.
- It is important to remember that both the researchers and the IRB members have a common goal: to advance the medical care of patients while protecting the subjects of those advancements.

FINANCIAL DISCLOSURE

The authors have nothing to disclose.

REFERENCES

1. "Nuremberg Code". The Doctor's Trial: The Medical Case of the Subsequent Nuremberg Proceedings. United States Holocaust Memorial Museum Online Exhibitions. Retrieved December 12th, 2022.
2. Zimbardo PG, Haney C, Banks WC, Jaffe D. The Stanford prison experiment, Zimbardo, Incorporated, 1971.
3. National Institutes of Health, The National Commission for the Protection of Human Subjects of Biomedical and Behavioral Research. The Belmont Report: ethical principles and guidelines for the protection of human subjects of research. 1979.
4. Moon MR, Khin-Maung-Gyi F. The history and role of institutional review boards. Virtual Mentor 2009;11(4):311–6.
5. 45 CFR Part 46. Available at: https://www.ecfr.gov/current/title-45/subtitle-A/subchapter-A/part-46. Accessed December 31, 2022.
6. Office for Human Research Protections. Reviewing and Reporting Unanticipated Problems Involving Risks to Subjects or Others and Adverse Events: OHRP Guidance, 2007. U.S. Department of Health & Human Services. https://www.hhs.gov/ohrp/regulations-and-policy/guidance/reviewing-unanticipated-problems/index.html#Q2. Accessed January 31, 2023.

Grants and Funding in Podiatric Science

Aksone Nouvong, DPM[a],*, Jessica Jaswal, DPM, MS[b],
David Aungst, DPM[a]

KEYWORDS

• Podiatric research • Podiatric surgery • Podiatry funding and grants

KEY POINTS

• Evidence-based research is integral to advance the field of podiatric medicine and surgery. It should be encouraged for young podiatric surgeon scientists.
• Interdisciplinary mentorship and collaboration provide a framework for grant procurement and research dissemination.
• There are several funding opportunities and grants available for podiatric research including, but not limited to, intramural, extramural, and governmental sources.
• It is essential to apply for grants and funding opportunities broadly, extensively, and early.

INTRODUCTION

Evidence-based medicine and research are the cornerstone for advancements in medicine and surgery. In the past century, only nine surgeons have been awarded the Nobel Prize, representing 5% of all recipients.[1,2] The discovery of vascular organ transplantation by Alexis Carrell, penicillin by Alexander Fleming, insulin by Frederick Banting, and the thyroid gland pathology by Theodor Kocher are just a few examples of such research that has transformed medicine and surgery through translational surgical application.[1–3] Given our work which entails extensive medical training, intimate knowledge of human anatomy and physiology, and hands-on experience, surgeon scientists are in a unique position to develop and conduct meaningful research with profound implications for clinical application but may encounter several barriers in this pursuit, such as procuring funding.[3]

Funding is one of the main determinants in scientific research and advancement.[4] Securing appropriate funds is essential in completing research projects and imperative for surgeon scientists, such as podiatric surgeons, or those conducting

---

[a] Department of Surgery, David Geffen School of Medicine at University of California, Los Angeles, Gonda Vascular Surgery, 200 Medical Plaza, Suite 504, Los Angeles, CA 90095, USA;
[b] PGY3, Department of Surgery, University of California, Los Angeles, Gonda Vascular Surgery, 200 Medical Plaza, Suite 504, Los Angeles, CA 90095, USA
* Corresponding author.
E-mail address: anouvong@mednet.ucla.edu

Clin Podiatr Med Surg 41 (2024) 247–257
https://doi.org/10.1016/j.cpm.2023.06.012
0891-8422/24/© 2023 Elsevier Inc. All rights reserved.

evidence-based research. Several barriers have been identified for surgeon scientists pursuing research such as the lack of funding, lack of dedicated research time and mentorship, and extensive clinical responsibilities.[3–7] However, the lack of securing funds has terminated many research projects and studies before they even begin. Furthermore, despite funding sources and grants being available, navigating through these resources is challenging and can be insurmountable for an early investigator.

It is known that research and discovery are a catalyst for improving science and human thinking and are a well-defined path to improving mankind.[1] Over the years, we have seen this be evident in podiatry. As we continue to publish peer-reviewed, evidence-based research, we not only continue to improve podiatric physician parity, but we provide patients with the most advanced and evidence-based lower extremity care. With 25% of the US population having diabetes, and diabetic foot ulcerations increasing morbidity by 85% while accounting for a national annual spending of $17 billions, the investment in podiatric research not only is cost-effective but also saves limbs and lives.[8–10] It is estimated that podiatric research and care can reduce the cost of diabetes-related complications in California alone by $97 million, which would further reduce the economic burden on an already fragile health care system.[8] Podiatric surgeon scientists have an integral role in the well-being of our health care system, and as such, we should continue to promote and conduct meaningful, evidence-based research. The goal of this article is to provide current information on the different types of grants and funding sources applicable for podiatric surgeon scientists.

DISCUSSION
Current State of Podiatric Research

Over the past 20 years, we have seen an exponential increase in 1-year foot and ankle fellowship programs.[11] Some of these fellowships programs are recognized by and closely monitored by the American College of Foot and Ankle Surgeons which has established mandatory surgical and academic objectives, including but not limited to evidence-based research. Although some residency programs promote resident-based research, fellowship programs often require research for successful matriculation. A recent study examined post-fellowship research productivity at 3, 5, and 10 years, demonstrating that despite the growing number of foot and ankle fellowships, only a small portion continue to publish research after completing fellowship and mainly only by individuals that work with university-based practices.[11] Although there are many factors in the decline of postgraduate foot and ankle research productivity within multispecialty groups or private practices compared with university-based employment, which may offer promotional incentives for research, access to funding and research grants should not be overlooked.[11] Rather, we believe that lack of funds is a major limitation in postgraduate publications, as navigating funding resources for podiatric physicians is challenging and ill-defined.

Essential components of funding

Many factors should be considered when procuring funds, but we believe there are three fundamental principles. First, recognize all potential funding sources available. Second, one should consider all applicable and unique funding opportunities based on the specific stage of their career. Funding opportunities change based on the progression of one's career, and it is imperative to be aware of these changes to maximize funds.[12] Finally, one should know of all grant requirements and timelines before grant submission.

The National Institutes of Health (NIH) is the main funding source for scientific research in the United States. However, over the past decade, it has become increasingly difficult to obtain NIH grants by surgeon scientists due to the increase in applicants and decrease in overall grants funded.[13] For successful funding and grant procurement, surgeon scientists need strong clinical and surgical mentorship to nurture their scientific interests, assist with grant writing, and obtain departmental support.

Grants for students, residents, and fellows

To instill the foundational importance of research, there are several societies and institutions that provide grant and funding opportunities for young professionals starting out their careers. A few such funding opportunities for young professionals in podiatric medicine and surgery to consider are student organizations, academic institutions and departments, research scholarships, and surgical societies. Applicants are typically required to be members of these societies and required to submit grant applications 6 months to 1 year before study initiation.[12] Although competitive, these funding sources are more attainable for surgeon scientists as they are intended to be training grants for professional development.[12–14] These grants require thorough study protocols, methodologies, timelines, budgetary requests, faculty mentorship, and a well-written grant application. They encourage critical thinking and provide young surgeon scientists advanced grant-writing experience. In addition, there are NIH grants for young surgical professionals such as the NIH T-series, or training grants, and the F-series, or fellowship training grants. These grants have rigorous requirements; however, they may provide salary and tuition support, which appeals to surgeon scientists as they balance their research and professional responsibilities.[12,15]

Grants for faculty

There are several intramural and extramural funding sources for faculty members participating in various capacities of research. A few such funding sources are institutional, philanthropic, foundational, medical and surgical societies, industry sponsors, and governmental agencies.

Intramural funding. Academic institutions may offer senate research grants, which are awarded annually and can be up to $10,000.[16] These funds do not carry over into new fiscal years and may have flexible budgetary terms depending on the allocation amount and academic institution. Departments within each academic institution also have grants and funding for faculty members and collaborators. Departments may require a written grant proposal that is reviewed by departmental research committees. These grants have rigorous timelines and requirements to prepare faculty members for larger grant applications. In addition, start-up funds or seed grants are designated funds for new faculty members allocated by an academic institution or department for research activities. These funds are typically dispersed in one large amount at the beginning of a faculty appointment or may be annually allocated over the course of several academic years. They can be negotiated based on faculty member research experience, interests, and the years of allocation requested.[12,15,17] Institutions may also provide career-development funding sources such as pilot funding or multi-year award mechanisms for certain research projects. These funding mechanisms are typically more flexible and can be annually renewed.

Extramural funding. Medical and surgical societies offer grants for surgeon scientists, a few of which are highlighted in **Box 1**. Theses societies have grants ranging from $25,000 to $100,000 with various stipulations, requirements, and financial support for 1 to 2 years. These grants can be used to fund a study or to augment start-up funds for higher budget projects. Applying for these smaller scale grants provides an

---

Box 1
Medical and surgical societies with funding opportunities most relevant to podiatric surgeon scientists

American Academy of Orthopaedic Surgeons

American Academy of Orthotists Prosthetists

American Association for the Surgery of Trauma

American Association for Women Podiatrists

American Association of Plastic Surgeons

American Burn Association

American College of Foot and Ankle Surgeons

American College of Surgeons

American Diabetes Association

American Orthopaedic Foot and Ankle Society

American Orthopaedic Society for Sports Medicine

American Orthotic and Prosthetics Association

American Podiatric Medical Association

American Podiatric Medical Students Association

American Public Health Association

American Surgical Association

Association of Women Surgeons

Center for Orthotic and Prosthetic Learning and Outcomes/Evidence Based Practice

Diabetes Research Connection

National Institute on Disability, Independent Living, and Rehabilitation Research

Orthopaedic Trauma Association

Orthotic and Prosthetic Education and Research Foundation

Pediatric Orthopaedic Society of North America

Society of Vascular Surgery

Surgical Infection Society

---

opportunity to improve grant-writing skills for larger, governmental grants and offers mentored support for researchers moving into the independent investigator phase.[12,18]

Private funding. Philanthropic or endowment funds should be explored as they typically do not have many research stipulations. These sources have allocated funds devoted to research initiatives or specific disease processes that align with the donors' interests such as limb salvage, nerve pathology, or traumatic injury. As such, these funds may have restricted or unrestricted terms depending on donor motivation and interest.[19] Similarly, foundational grants are private funding sources that have dedicated funds for research dedicated to certain disease processes or specific demographics. Foundation committees generally compromise of non-scientific, non-medical board members who have an intimate relationship with a disease or research initiative. As such, it is recommended that grant proposals use laymen terms to convey research goals in a clear and concise manner.

Other means of research funding is through industry or pharmaceutical sponsored grants. This type of funding is sponsored by an organization to conduct clinical trials that may involve an intervention or observation of a disease or condition. For surgical specialties that work closely with medical technology companies, there is opportunity to conduct sponsored or funded research. Often, the research is aligned with the mutual interest of the surgeon scientists and the objectives of the products or technologies offered by the companies, such as pressure injuries, prevention of surgical site infections, implant efficacies, or hospital-acquired infections.[20] This type of funded research may pose conflict of interest and conflict with rights to research and may have potential bias. Project proposals and grant applications are sent to the medical technology company 6 months to 1 year in advance.

Governmental Agency Funding

There are 26 different federal agencies and several independent agencies, executive branch offices, and commissions that offer research grants applicable to podiatric physicians and surgeon scientists. Although independent agencies may offer grants with a smaller budget than those directly from federal executive departments, it is recommended to explore all funding options. A few agencies are highlighted in **Box 2** but also include the US Department of Health and Human Services, US Department of

---

Box 2
Foundations and agencies with funding opportunities most relevant to podiatric surgeon scientists

Agency for Health Research and Quality

AO Foundation

Arthritis Foundation

Center for Disease Control

Kaiser Permanente

Melanoma Institute of Health

National Institute of Health

National Science Foundation

Orthopaedic Research and Education Foundation

Patient-Centered Outcomes and Research Institute

The Gates Foundation

The National Institute of Diabetes and Digestive and Kidney Diseases

United States Department of Defense Congressionally Directed Medical Research Programs

United States Department of Veterans Affairs (VA) Office of Research and Development

United States Government Grants

University of California Discovery Grant

University of California Research Initiatives

Urgo Foundation

World Diabetes Foundation

Wound Healing Foundation

Veterans Affairs, Agency for Healthcare Research and Quality, the Centers of Disease Control and Prevention, and Patient-Centered Outcomes Research Institute.[21]

Roadmap to NIH grants

The NIH comprises of 27 institutes and centers, 24 of which contribute to grant awards that support research. There are separate funding appropriations from Congress, and the director of each institute reserves the jurisdiction to determine which grants to fund.[15] The NIH provides financial support in the form of independent grants, cooperative agreements, career development awards, and loan repayment funding sources. For most independent grants, the NIH uses a project period system through which a project undergoes a peer review process and, if approved, will receive funding in annual increments for up to 5 years. Budgetary requests and allocations for NIH grants are more flexible than institutional grants as one can incorporate a stipend for faculty mentorship, research resources, and publication expenses, ultimately allowing for devoted research time. There are several grant mechanisms within the NIH applicable to podiatric surgeon scientists such as the R, T, K, and F grants, and there are three annual award cycles for these grants.[15] Although NIH grants are difficult to obtain without prior grant awards and are often a barrier to surgeon scientists pursuing funding, they are attainable but require perseverance and an aptitude for research.

The NIH R-series

There are several R-series grants that are applicable to podiatric surgeons, some of which we will highlight. These grants may be awarded to universities, hospital, research institutes, or health care professionals that conduct biomedical research and development.[15] The NIH R01, or investigator-initiated research project grant, is the original, eldest, and most commonly used NIH grant mechanism. It is considered the "gold standard" of independent research grants and is funded by all institutes of the NIH.[12,13] The R01 grants are competitive yet highly prestigious with an acceptance funding rate of 10%. These grants support research projects for 3 to 5 years and can be renewed.[12,15,22] This mechanism does not have a specific funding limit and typically awards a $250,000 annual modular budget; however, for funding requests over $500,000, advanced permission from the NIH with budgetary justification can be requested.[12] These grants do not have funding stipulations and provide recipients the freedom to allocate funds as they see appropriate for research purposes. These grants may be used for salaries, research equipment and supplies, travel, and other direct or indirect research costs.[15,22]

There are additional R-series grants, not funded by all institutes of the NIH, that can provide funding for small-scale research studies. These mechanisms are not meant to be in lieu of an R01 but are rather meant for distinct, focused, research studies that do not qualify for a traditional R01. The R03, or small grant program, is a non-renewable grant mechanism that provides limited annual funding of $50,000 for a 2-year period to support various projects including pilot or feasibility studies, collection of preliminary data, secondary analysis of existing data, or for the development of new research methodologies or technologies. The R15, or academic research enhancement award, is a multi-year award which provides up to $300,000 over a project 3-year period. This grant is defined by supporting small-scale research projects conducted by graduate students or faculty that have not been recipients of major NIH research grants. This grant mechanism is favorable as it supports meritorious research, exposes graduate students and young surgeon scientists to research, and builds their portfolio of awards and grants.[15] The R21, or exploratory research grant award, provides funding up to $275,000 for a project period of 2 years. It is directed to support exploratory or developmental research projects with high risk which may lead to breakthrough findings or the development of novel techniques that can have a major impact in clinical research.[12–15]

Supplemental NIH series

The NIH offers K-series, T-series, and F-series grants. The K-series, or career-development awards, are clinical-scientist and patient-care oriented awards. These grants (K01, K02, K08, K12, K23) provide residents, fellows, and surgeon scientists an opportunity to apply for an NIH-level grant with flexible requirements and budgets. This grant is awarded to establish research laboratories and clinical investigation under a senior mentor.[13] Recently, the number of K-series to R01-level award conversions has been uptrending among surgical specialties.[13] The T-series (T32, T35), or Ruth L Kirschstein Institutional National Research Service Awards (NRSA), and the F-series, or Ruth L Kirschstein Individual NRSA (F31, F21, F33), are grants that can be awarded to an institution or individuals at various levels of their careers for specific research initiatives and should be explored for podiatric research funding.

To successfully procure grants, one should be aware of all policies and initiatives that may be beneficial for their funding goals. One such policy is the Early Stage Investigator (ESI) status offered by the NIH. An ESI is a principal investigator who has either completed their terminal research degree or completed their postgraduate/residency/fellowship training within the past 10 years and has not been awarded an NIH independent research award, such as an R01 or R01 equivalent.[15] Being a recipient of a smaller grant such as the K, T, or F series does not affect ones ESI status or eligibility. By using ESI status, a grant application receives special consideration during the review and funding process by being allocated an impact score and percentile ranking. There is also a distinct payline for ESIs by each NIH institute, funding up to ten percentile points higher than the standard R01 payline.[12,15] In addition, reviewers may allow exceptions for less-impactful publications and data for grants submitted under ESI. Another mechanism of building a portfolio with the NIH is through the loan repayment programs (LRPs). The LRPs are organized around broad research areas and are not intended to fund a specific research project. It is designed to recruit and retain health professionals to pursue NIH-relevant research by repaying $50,000 annually for 2 years of a researcher's educational debt. The LRPs are an attractive and relevant program for surgeon scientists and young podiatric providers as patient work can be easily demonstrated, while building a record of research with the NIH. Applying through the ESI status and LRP program are a few methods of being an assiduous researcher and creating a robust track record of successful NIH funding procurement.

Department of defense

The United States Department of Defense Congressionally Directed Medical Research Programs (CDMRP) is another avenue of research funding for podiatric surgeons. The CDMRP was established via congressional appropriations to foster novel research and manage research programs focused on diseases, injuries, and topic areas directed by Congress. The CDMRP is known to fund high-impact, high-risk, and high-reward research projects that other governmental agencies may not fund. One program funded by the CDMRP which is relevant to podiatric surgeon scientists with aims to improve quality of life for patients with lower extremity injuries and disabilities is the Orthotics and Prosthetics Outcomes Program (OPORP). The OPORP receives $10 million of Congressional appropriations annually to facilitate orthotic and prosthetic device implementation and offers clinical trial and clinical research awards for research to advance device form, device fit, and device function.[23] The program has a multidisciplinary panel which reviews grant applications by a peer-review two-tier system and encourages podiatric physicians to apply.[23]

Summary

Although funding is not necessary to conduct meaningful, evidence-based research, funds can help offset the cost of research, participant involvement, and supplies/equipment and allow for dedicated research personnel time and resources. It is imperative to be cognizant of all relevant and applicable grants, funding sources, and unique subcategories such as wound care, trauma, sports medicine, or orthotics and prosthetics to optimize funding opportunities. Identifying funding sources will equip one with the highest funding procurement rate. It is also crucial to explore funding sources from each tier of the funding pyramid (**Fig. 1**). This pyramid provides a framework for grants that are attainable based on one's capacity of research experience, portfolio of grant procurements, and overall project needs. For instance, obtaining an NIH award is regarded as one of the most prestigious and coveted grants given the rigorous application and vetting process. An applicant that has received prior NIH funding, an R01, or R01 equivalent grant, is regarded as a strong applicant and is more likely

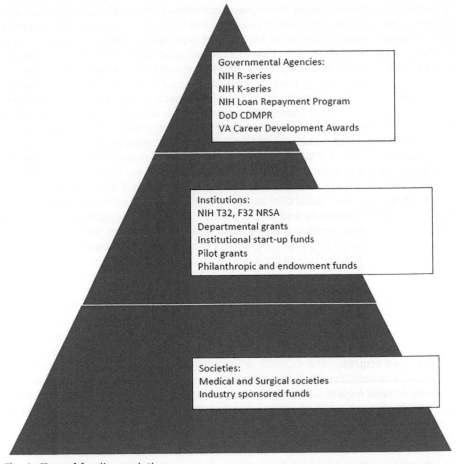

Governmental Agencies:
NIH R-series
NIH K-series
NIH Loan Repayment Program
DoD CDMPR
VA Career Development Awards

Institutions:
NIH T32, F32 NRSA
Departmental grants
Institutional start-up funds
Pilot grants
Philanthropic and endowment funds

Societies:
Medical and Surgical societies
Industry sponsored funds

Fig. 1. Tiers of funding societies.

to procure governmental agency funding in the future. However, a young surgeon scientist that has not been awarded prior governmental funding should build their portfolio with smaller agency grants and institutional awards. Given the barriers for surgeon scientists to obtain funding, it is recommended to apply for smaller, attainable grants and move up to NIH R-level funding sources.

Once appropriate grants and funding sources have been identified, it is essential to begin the grant-writing process. It is recommended to contact each grant program officer before submission to ensure that the grant mechanism is appropriate for the applicant and research study. It is then imperative to establish a multidisciplinary, core team of mentors and collaborators with a wide breadth of research experience to assist with grant writing, project management, grant submissions, outlining a roadmap for deadlines, and assisting with the dissemination of research outcomes. Having a network of diverse collaborators, including health care professionals and academics, provides access to funding opportunities and specialized resources that may not otherwise be available.

Writing a research proposal is an arduous and rigorous process that may require multiple proposal iterations before submission. It is encouraged to use institutional resources for assistance with grant writing, budget preparation, proposal review, and grant submission. It is important to stay within the parameters of the grant requirements and provide a strong proposal with a well-defined budget, considering every aspect of the research study that may require financial input.[24,25] As with all advice, we recommend applying early, at least 6 months to 1 year before project start, and applying often. There are several pitfalls in the grant-writing and application processes that should be avoided.

COMMON PITFALLS

- Lack of knowledge on applicable grants, funding parameters, and sources.
- Lack of organization in terms of budget requests, letters of support, and timeline of deliverables.
- Not applying broadly and categorically for grants.
- Not applying for grants early and often. Initially, there will be more rejections than acceptances, and persistence is essential.
- Not incorporating reviewer feedback into grant resubmissions.
- Lack of interdisciplinary collaboration and mentorship.

Evidence-based research is imperative to advancing the field of podiatric medicine and surgery. The pursuit of research for surgeon scientists is met with many barriers, the greatest of which is funding. Although challenging, this can be traversed by leveraging extramural and intramural institutional support and strong mentorship. This article presents a roadmap to guide podiatric research funding and demonstrates funding is attainable and should be encouraged.

CLINICS CARE POINTS

- Evidence-based research is essential to advance podiatric medicine and surgery.
- Apply early, apply often. Grants require a significant investment of time, energy, and effort.
- Apply for grants with a smaller budget and scope to build a funding portfolio, before applying for larger governmental grants.
- Mentorship, collaboration, and networking are critical in grant procurement.

- Ensure research applications can be translated into clinical practice and policy.

DISCLOSURE

The authors have nothing to disclose.

REFERENCES

1. Toledo-Pereyra LH. Nobel laureate surgeons. J Invest Surg 2006;19(4):211–8.
2. Kanematsu T. The happy marriage of surgery and science/technology would lead to prosperous surgical development towards the year 2050. Surg Today 2010; 40(8):691–5.
3. Livingston-Rosanoff D, Park KY, Alagoz E, Thibeault S, Gibson A. Setting up for success: strategies to foster surgeons' pursuit of basic science research. J Surg Res 2021;268:71–8.
4. Ebadi A, Schiffauerova A. How to receive more funding for your research? Get connected to the right people. PLoS One 2015;10(7):e0133061.
5. Kodadek LM, Kapadia MR, Changoor NR, et al. Educating the surgeon-scientist: a qualitative study evaluating challenges and barriers toward becoming an academically successful surgeon. Surgery 2016;160(6):1456–65.
6. Keswani SG, Moles CM, Morowitz M, et al. The future of basic science in academic surgery: identifying barriers to success for surgeon-scientists. Ann Surg 2017;265(6):1053–9.
7. Goldstein AM, Blair AB, Keswani SG, et al. A roadmap for aspiring surgeon-scientists in today's healthcare environment. Ann Surg 2019;269(1):66–72.
8. Toledo-Pereyra LH. Importance of medical and surgical research. J Invest Surg 2009;22(5):325–6.
9. Labovitz J, Kominski GF, Godwin J. Podiatric services could reduce costs of treating diabetes complications in California by up to $97 Million. eScholarship, University of California. Available at: https://escholarship.org/uc/item/4f75k8d1. Published May 8, 2018. Accessed January 02, 2023.
10. Brownrigg JR, Davey J, Holt PJ, et al. The association of ulceration of the foot with cardiovascular and all-cause mortality in patients with diabetes: a meta-analysis. Diabetologia 2012;55(11):2906–12.
11. Barshes NR, Sigireddi M, Wrobel JS, et al. The system of care for the diabetic foot: objectives, outcomes, and opportunities. Diabet Foot Ankle 2013;4. https://doi.org/10.3402/dfa.v4i0.21847.
12. Casciato DJ, Thompson J, Hyer CF. Post-fellowship foot and ankle surgeon research productivity: a systematic review. J Foot Ankle Surg 2022;61(4):896–9.
13. Gosain A, Chu DI, Smith JJ, Neuman HB, Goldstein AM, Zuckerbraun BS. Climbing the grants ladder: funding opportunities for surgeons. Surgery 2021;170(3):707–12.
14. Narahari AK, Mehaffey JH, Hawkins RB, et al. Surgeon scientists are disproportionately affected by declining NIH funding rates. J Am Coll Surg 2018;226(4):474–81.
15. Mansukhani NA, Patti MG, Kibbe MR. Rebranding "the lab years" as "professional development" in order to redefine the modern surgeon scientist. Ann Surg 2017; 266(6):937–8.
16. Grants & Funding. National Institutes of Health. Available at: https://www.nih.gov/grants-funding. Accessed January 02, 2023.

17. Cor Faculty Grants Program: Research Grants. Academic Senate. Available at: https://senate.ucla.edu/committee/cor/fgp. Published December 15, 2022. Accessed January 02, 2023.
18. Early career research funding opportunities: Research & innovation. University of Nevada, Reno. Available at: https://www.unr.edu/research-innovation/research-hub/early-career. Accessed January 02, 2023.
19. Gift vs grant. Gift vs Grant. Available at: https://hcsra.sph.harvard.edu/gift-vs-grant. Accessed January 02, 2023.
20. Emamaullee J, Lian T, Moroz S, Zuckerbraun B, Matthews J, Gosain A. Defining the "tipping point" to success as a surgeon-scientist: an analysis of applicants and awardees of the American college of surgeons Jacobson promising investigator award. Ann Surg 2022;275(5):e678–82.
21. Pickles S, Kiel-Monaghan I. Stryker Clinical Research. Stryker. Available at: https://www.strykermeded.com/education/stryker-clinical-research/. Accessed January 03, 2023.
22. Find. apply. succeed. GRANTS.GOV. Available at: https://www.grants.gov/web/grants/learn-grants/grant-programs.html. Accessed January 03, 2023.
23. Mitchell E. Why are R01 NIH grants such a big deal? Health.Care. Available at: https://blog.eoscu.com/blog/why-are-r01-nih-grants-such-a-big-deal. Published January 5, 2022. Accessed January 03, 2023.
24. Transforming healthcare through innovative and Impactful Research. Orthotics and Prosthetics Outcomes Research Program, Congressionally Directed Medical Research Programs. Available at: https://cdmrp.health.mil/oporp/default. Accessed January 03, 2023.
25. Cleary M, Walter G, Hunt G. The quest to fund research: playing research lotto. Australas Psychiatry 2006;14(3):323–6.

A New Paradigm in Foot and Ankle Outcomes?
Away From Radiographs and Toward Patient-Centered Outcomes

Naohiro Shibuya, DPM, MS, FACFAS[a],*,
Monica R. Agarwal, DPM, FACFAS[a], Daniel C. Jupiter, PhD[b]

KEYWORDS

- Reliability • Validity • Patient-reported outcome • Radiographic measures
- Patient-centered care

KEY POINTS

- Patient-centered care is becoming more valued.
- Patient-reported outcome measures (PROMs) are, therefore, becoming more common in clinical research.
- Reasonable outcome measures must have sound reliability, validity, efficacy, and responsiveness but lack the ceiling and floor effects.
- Provider-measured outcomes, such as radiographic measures, are becoming less valued because of the potential lack of reliability and correlation with PROMs.

INTRODUCTION

Research should bring us closer to the truth. Knowing the truth is the ultimate goal of science; nevertheless, this aim is unattainable, as we cannot possibly account for every variable in the universe. Therefore, we must settle for less-than-perfect research methodologies. However, this does not mean that research should be disregarded altogether; in fact, quite the opposite is true, as a well-controlled study will always improve our understanding of the world.

In many scientific disciplines, objective analysis of the matter at hand is essential. However, in medical research, subjective inputs from patients are also important, as the most important goal of medical research is to improve the well-being of the patients. In foot and ankle research, the quality of patients' lives, treatment efficacy,

[a] University of Texas Rio Grande Valley, School of Podiatric Medicine; [b] Department of Biostatistics and Data Science, Orthopaedic Surgery and Rehabilitation, The University of Texas Medical Branch, 2101 Treasure Hills Boulevard, Harlingen, TX 78550, USA
* Corresponding author.
E-mail address: naohiro.shibuya@utrgv.edu

Clin Podiatr Med Surg 41 (2024) 259–268
https://doi.org/10.1016/j.cpm.2023.06.013
0891-8422/24/© 2023 Elsevier Inc. All rights reserved.

and procedure safety should improve through better understanding of the procedure, patients' bodies, and patients themselves. For years, foot and ankle research focused on the procedures and patients' bodies. However, the recent movement toward patient-centered care has shifted the focus toward patient-reported outcomes (PROs).[1] Instead of only reporting provider-measured outcomes (such as radiographic measurements), the trend is to capture outcomes from the patient's perspective. This shift in paradigm, and the advantages/disadvantages of this trend are discussed.

TYPES OF OUTCOME MEASURES COMMONLY USED IN FOOT AND ANKLE RESEARCH

Scientific reasoning requires the formulation of a hypothesis and the testing of that hypothesis. Outcome measures are needed to detect significant findings formulated in those hypotheses. Ideal outcome measures are free of errors and biases, they should be valid and reliable, and they should also be responsive to changes and not have floor or ceiling effects. From a practical standpoint, they should also be easy to use, reproducible, cost-effective for the investigators, and minimally cumbersome for the patients.

Error in measurement causes inaccurate results, and some outcome measures are more prone to measurement error than others. For example, measurements of Kite's angle in the dorsoplantar view of a plain radiograph of a foot can be subject to measurement error due to difficulty seeing the outlines of the talus and calcaneus and judging the axis of the corresponding osseous structures. On the other hand, measurements of the first intermetatarsal angle are much more straightforward, with more visible long bones. This type of disparity in measurement accuracy can cause inconsistency in study results, and one needs to be aware of this phenomenon.

An outcome measure also needs to be responsive to changes and free of floor or ceiling effects. Potentially, for example, a positive result, such as improved pain, can be lost when an investigator classifies pain into two broad dichotomized categories. Specifically, if preoperative and postoperative pain are measured as "yes" or "no," the broad spectrum of pain is lost in the dichotomized data. Similarly, the floor and ceiling effect of a measure can mask a potentially detectible difference between groups when the results are clustered in the maximum or minimum scores of the measure. For example, no difference can be detected among top students when an examination is too easy and when many students get 100% in the class. This ceiling effect does not prove that there is no difference between the top students, but rather makes the difference undetectable.

Validity refers to how well an outcome measure represents what is intended to be measured. For example, a patient's quality of life is often measured by scores obtained from surveys. How accurately the score represents patients' quality of life determines the validity of the survey instrument.

The validity of outcome measures is often overlooked in study design. A newly designed survey instrument must undergo vigorous validation processes to show relevance to the study question. The new instrument is said to be validated if the outcomes correlate well with previously validated instruments. Results obtained from unvalidated instruments may be inaccurate and may not answer the intended study question.

For the practicality of conducting research, cost-effectiveness and ease of use are also important. Often surgical outcome studies are conducted with patients filling out multiple surveys for PRO measures. This can take a great deal of time and create fatigue for patients, and the results can be inaccurate. From the perspective of patients and the survey administrator, an ideal instrument should be short, easy to use or read, and free of cultural bias.

CLINICIAN-BASED VERSUS PROs

Outcome measures can be categorized into provider-based and patient-centered measures (**Table 1**). Provider-based measures are independent of patients' feelings, opinions, and perspectives. Examples of these in foot and ankle research include radiographic angles, nonunion rate, and gait analysis. On the other hand, patient-centered measures are reported by patients and are independent of provider-based measures. These include patient satisfaction, pain, and quality of life, all reported via survey.

RADIOGRAPHIC MEASUREMENTS

It is common to study surgical outcomes in terms of radiographic measurements, namely angles, distances, and presence or absence of nonunion. While these measures have been considered clinically significant by clinicians, providers, and surgeons, they are not a direct measure of patients' perceived clinical outcomes. In fact, many studies have failed to show a relationship between PROs and radiographic measurements.[18,19] In such cases, one should question the importance of the radiographic measurements, as these measurements do not represent patients' perceived quality of medical/surgical treatments, and thus do not appear to impact patient outcomes.

Radiographic measurements can also be prone to measurement error. When the margin of error is greater than the detectable difference, the result is said to be

Table 1
Examples, pros, and cons of patient-reported outcomes versus provider-measured outcomes

	Patient-Reported Outcomes	Provider-Measured Outcomes
Pros	• Outcomes are patient-centered • More accepted in today's clinical research and practice	• More objective • Convenient for investigators
Cons	• More subjective • Often not specific enough • May be cumbersome for patients • May be costly	• Do not incorporate patients' perspective • May not have any clinical significance
Examples	• Patient-Reported Outcomes Measure Instrument Systems (PROMIS)[2,3] • Visual Analogue Score (VAS) for pain[4] • 36-Item Short Form Health Survey (SF-36)[5] • Foot and Ankle Ability Measure (FAAM) Score[6] • Foot and Ankle Outcome Score (FAOS)[7] • EuroQol EQ-5D[8] • Foot Function Index (FFI)[9] • Self-reported Foot and Ankle Score (SEFAS)[10] • Western Ontario and McMaster (WOMAC) Osteoarthritis Index Score[11] • Short Musculoskeletal Function Assessment (SMFA) Questionnaire[12] • Ankle Osteoarthritis Scale (AOS)[13]	• Radiographic measures • Gait analysis • Manual muscle testing[14] • Nonunion rate • Range of motion • American College of Foot and Ankle Surgeons (ACFAS) score[15] • American Orthopaedic Foot and Ankle Society (AOFAS) score[16] • Olerud-Molander Ankle Score • Japanese Society for Surgery of the Foot (JSSF)[17]

inaccurate. Measurement errors can stem from a measurement method, a rater's experience, the anatomical location at which the measure is taken, or the type of measurement, as detailed in the following sections.

Using manual instruments such as a ruler, caliper, tractograph, or goniometer on plain x-ray films was common in the past to measure the angles and distances. While the manual instruments themselves may be precise, an error can be introduced by the users of the instruments. These methods can be improved in terms of accuracy with computer measurement systems with or without additional software.[20–22]

Even with accurate tools, there are issues with points of reference and the definitions of radiographic measurements.[23] Location, position, and type of structures being measured can also greatly affect the accuracy of the results.[24,25] Reference points are often inconsistent between the observers and studies.[26,27] For example, "bisection of long bone" can be determined by different methods, by different observers, and in different studies. Such variability is often more prevalent in smaller, shorter long bones than in more easily visible long bones. Even in the case of a well-visualized anatomical structure, reference points can be subject to inaccuracy due to parallax created by the radiographic projection angle and distance.[28–30] Reduction of the 3-dimensional image into 2-dimensional measurements, therefore, can lead to discrepancy and inaccuracy.[31] Three-dimesnional CT scans and MRI measurements are often used to minimize this issue.[32–34]

The experience of the raters can also affect the measurements. The variability between raters is often mitigated by training them to standardize their definitions and methods of taking particular measurements before a research project begins. Alternately, taking an average of measurements made by different raters can neutralize errors created among the raters. Without these quality measures and assurances that the measures are of high quality, the results obtained from radiographic measurements can be unreliable. To show a result's reliability, many investigators evaluate interrater and intrarater reliabilities.[35,36] Analysis using measurements with poor interreliability and intrareliability should be questioned.

Another popular outcome measure in foot and ankle surgical research is the occurrence of nonunion. This, too, is not a direct measure of a clinical outcome from the patient's perspective, but it is more closely related to clinical symptoms, such as pain and satisfaction, than radiographic measures. It is, however, still prone to measurement error and inconsistency.[37] Many of the criteria within the definition of nonunion are subjective and prone to bias. Definitions of nonunion have different dimensions: It is a function of bone healing (often assessed by radiographs), time, and clinical symptoms.

Assessing nonunion on plain films can be subjective; poor-quality radiographs, an overlap of osseous structures, and soft-tissue edema often block the view and make judging key features such as cortical bridging challenging. While adjusting exposure and tone can improve visibility in a digital image, these improvements have their limits. Multiple views of plain radiographs are also used to minimize the aforementioned problem. Also, CT scan has been shown to be more reliable in identifying nonunions.

Time is a significant component in defining nonunions. Many studies define nonunion as a radiographically visible fusion/fracture site at the "final" visit, yet such studies may not have consistent follow-up times for all their subjects. This variability in follow-up length can bias the results: The shorter the follow-up, the more likely it is that "nonunion" is detected. For example, those with 10-year follow-up will more likely have union than those with only 3 months of follow-up.

Pain is often associated with nonunions; therefore, some use this symptom as part of the nonunion definition. However, it is often unclear in an article how authors dealt with contradicting results between the radiographic and the clinical signs. Often, conjunctions such as "AND" and "OR" in the definition of nonunion are not used correctly. If nonunion is defined by having the radiographic finding "AND" the clinical symptom, both these findings are needed to capture nonunion. If the radiographic finding "OR" the symptom is positive, only one of these findings is needed.

OTHER COMMONLY USED MEASURES IN FOOT AND ANKLE SURGERY

Biomechanical analysis (ie, range of motion and gait analysis) and time to return to work/activity are commonly used measures that are primarily based on providers' perspectives. These measures are also subject to measurement error. Averaging multiple attempts for a range of motion and gait analysis are common ways to minimize measurement errors. Return to work/activity, while important to many patients, is subject to the investigator's bias. If the investigator/surgeon has control over when the patient returns to a certain activity, the finding can be highly subjective and prone to bias. Further questions have been raised as to whether the measure is inherently biased.[38]

While many studies evaluate multiple outcomes, including these provider-based outcomes and PROs, in the same cohort, the correlation between these provider-based measures and PROs is rarely studied. The assumption is that the more physiological the gait and range of motion are and the quicker the return to activity, the better the PROs. However, the association many times is not present or simply has not been evaluated.

PATIENT-REPORTED OUTCOME MEASURES

The movement towards patient-centered care has significantly increased the utility of patient-reported outcome measures (PROMs). In the research setting, the patient's perceptions of and satisfaction with treatment outcomes are recorded via a survey form and quantified with a validated scale. The survey often gives a "score," and the number is used for statistical analysis. A broader categorization, for example, of satisfaction as "very satisfied," "satisfied," or "somewhat satisfied," is becoming less popular, as these can be subject to floor and ceiling effects, unresponsiveness, and validation issues.

In contrast, however, more sophisticated scoring systems are time-consuming, expensive, and cumbersome for patients even though they can provide more reliable, responsive results. Especially when subjects fill out multiple long surveys, they can become fatigued and thus potentially provide inaccurate answers.

The PROMs can also be vague and not specific to the pathology or treatment of interest. General questions in some PROMs may not relate to foot and ankle-specific issues. This generalization might result in unresponsive scores, inaccuracy, and difficulty detecting significant results. In these cases, the lack of significant results should not be treated as an absence of proof; instead, they indicate that more specific instruments are needed.

Patient-reported outcomes measurement information systems (PROMIS) were created to solve many issues often associated with cumbersome survey instruments. The National Institute of Health developed the system to capture different dimensions of outcomes from patients' perspectives while keeping it user-friendly and relatively short and maintaining validity. It uses many validated, relevant questions to obtain information from patients. The survey is designed so that the set of questions changes depending on the patient's response, minimizing the number of questions being asked.

The PROMIS has different versions for specific topics. It is available in multiple languages, each validated for cultural adaptation. It is also technologically easy to use and can be administered with minimum effort, for example, on a tablet while waiting for a provider.

The American Orthopaedic Foot and Ankle Society recommended that this instrument be used in foot and ankle research in their position statement in 2018.[39] Specifically, they support the use of the Physical Function Computerized Adaptive Test and Lower Extremity Computerized Adaptive Test. Along with PROMIS, they advocated for Foot and Ankle Ability Measure and Foot and Ankle Outcome Score (FAOS).

ASSOCIATION BETWEEN PROVIDER-BASED AND PATIENT-CENTERED OUTCOME MEASURES

Currently, in the practice of medicine, patient-centered measures are weighed more heavily than provider-based measures. However, in research, different study questions call for different measures. Therefore, both provider-based and patient-centered measures have their own scientific merits. Any foot and ankle procedure can be researched with either type of outcome measure. However, if the investigator is a clinician involved with a patient's medical/surgical care, identifying associations between provider-based and patient-centered measures should be of interest. For example, identifying an association between postoperative hallux valgus angle and PROs should be interesting for surgeons to judge the usefulness of the objective measure in future treatment and research.

Matthews and colleagues[19] investigated the correlation between radiographic measurements and patient-centered outcomes in hallux valgus surgery. They tested the FAOS subscale scores against radiographic measurements such as postoperative hallux valgus angle, intermetatarsal angles, and metatarsal protrusion. They mostly did not find significant correlations between these measures. This finding is interesting, as this result leads us to infer that surgeons could have been focusing on surgically improving those radiographic measures, even though they did not matter to the patients. With this lack of correlation, the traditional focus in hallux valgus surgery might need to be re-evaluated.

Several reasons exist for the lack of association between provider-based outcomes and PROs. First, the relationship may, indeed, not exist. Improving the hallux valgus angle may not improve PROs, and surgeons may need to re-evaluate the paradigm altogether. Second, the method by which the relationship was assessed is not adequate. The inaccuracy of either type of measurement can mask associations. Alternatively, sometimes the relationship exists but is not necessarily a linear relationship; standard statistical tools may not detect it. While intermetatarsal angle as a continuous variable may not correlate with a PRO score, a range of values (ie, hallux valgus angle of <9 degrees) may. Third, other factors not accounted for in the study can influence the relationship of interest. For example, PROs may not be associated with nonunions in an arthrodesis study with many diabetic neuropathic patients, but the relationship may become apparent when the neuropathic patients are excluded.

On the other hand, there are many instances where PROs are associated with provider-based measurements. Shibuya and colleagues[40] showed a correlation between the modified ACFAS Rearfoot (Module 3) score and the 36-item short form version 2.0 (SF-36 v2). The ACFAS scale has multiple radiographic measures, while the SF-36 measures patient-reported quality of life. The combination of the radiographic measure was associated with the patient's perceived quality of life in the study. Therefore, a surgeon may be able to improve a patient's quality of life by improving the components in the ACFAS scale.

Finding the association between provider-based measures and PROs will be essential in future medical research. Objective measures need to be evaluated against clinically relevant measures, including PROs.

SUMMARY
The Future

Patient-centered care will continue to grow, and medical research will focus more on patients' perspectives. For this reason, results and conclusions stemming from PROs will be valued and used in policymaking and by insurance companies more often in the future. At the same time, we cannot completely disregard provider-based measures because we need these measures to understand the science and to identify factors associated with improving PROs. At the same time, a lack of association between provider-based and patient-centered measures will more likely result in a reevaluation of provider-perceived outcome measures than in that of patient-centered ones. On the other hand, identifying these associations would confirm the importance of the objective measures and enable the providers to better manage patients by improving these specific parameters.

PROs will be more widely incorporated not only in medical/surgical research but also in daily clinical practice. Patients will become accustomed to filling out short item-response surveys more often. The results of these surveys will be available for the physician as feedback and as a tool to communicate with the patients.

Provider-based measures should continue to be vetted for validity and reliability. Those provider-based measures strongly correlated with PROs are more likely to be refined and used further in medical research. Those measures with poor quality or association with PROs will become less popular, and studies using these measures will have a more challenging time being accepted by clinical journals.

CLINICS CARE POINTS

- Recognize that PROs are becoming the standard.
- Avoid focusing only on provider-based measures.
- Evaluate the relationships between PROs and provider-based measures.

POINTS OF INTEREST

- More medical/surgical journals will look for studies using outcome measures from the patient's perspective.
- When provider-based measures are used, many medical/surgical journals will expect to see the relationship of these objective measures to PROs.
- Health care systems and insurance companies will focus more on reviewing clinical studies tied to PROs for policymaking.

DISCLOSURE

The authors have nothing to disclose.

REFERENCES

1. Hunt KJ, Lakey E. Patient-reported outcomes in foot and ankle surgery. Orthop Clin North Am 2018;49(2):277–89.
2. Hung M, Baumhauer JF, Licari FW, et al. Responsiveness of the PROMIS and FAAM instruments in foot and ankle orthopedic population. Foot Ankle Int 2019; 40(1):56–64.
3. Nixon DC, McCormick JJ, Johnson JE, et al. PROMIS pain interference and physical function scores correlate with the foot and ankle ability measure (FAAM) in patients with hallux valgus. Clin Orthop Relat Res 2017;475(11):2775–80.
4. Wessel J. The reliability and validity of pain threshold measurements in osteoarthritis of the knee. Scand J Rheumatol 1995;24(4):238–42.
5. Hays RD, Sherbourne CD, Mazel RM. The RAND 36-item health survey 1.0. Health Econ 1993;2(3):217–27.
6. Martin RL, Irrgang JJ, Burdett RG, et al. Evidence of validity for the foot and ankle ability measure (FAAM). Foot Ankle Int 2005;26(11):968–83.
7. Roos EM, Brandsson S, Karlsson J. Validation of the foot and ankle outcome score for ankle ligament reconstruction. Foot Ankle Int 2001;22(10):788–94.
8. Svensson E. Construction of a single global scale for multi-item assessments of the same variable. Stat Med 2001;20(24):3831–46.
9. Budiman-Mak E, Conrad KJ, Roach KE. The foot function index: a measure of foot pain and disability. J Clin Epidemiol 1991;44(6):561–70.
10. Coster M, Karlsson MK, Nilsson JA, et al. Validity, reliability, and responsiveness of a self-reported foot and ankle score (SEFAS). Acta Orthop 2012;83(2): 197–203.
11. Bellamy N, Buchanan WW, Goldsmith CH, et al. Validation study of WOMAC: a health status instrument for measuring clinically important patient relevant outcomes to antirheumatic drug therapy in patients with osteoarthritis of the hip or knee. J Rheumatol 1988;15(12):1833–40.
12. Swiontkowski MF, Engelberg R, Martin DP, et al. Short musculoskeletal function assessment questionnaire: validity, reliability, and responsiveness. J Bone Joint Surg Am 1999;81(9):1245–60.
13. Domsic RT, Saltzman CL. Ankle osteoarthritis scale. Foot Ankle Int 1998;19(7): 466–71.
14. Council MR. Special report series no 282. London, UK: Her Majesty's Stationery Office; 1954. p. 64–72.
15. Thomas JL, Christensen JC, Mendicino RW, et al. ACFAs scoring scale user guide. J Foot Ankle Surg 2005;44(5):316–35.
16. Kitaoka HB, Alexander IJ, Adelaar RS, et al. Clinical rating systems for the ankle-hindfoot, midfoot, hallux, and lesser toes. Foot Ankle Int 1994;15(7):349–53.
17. Niki H, Aoki H, Inokuchi S, et al. Development and reliability of a standard rating system for outcome measurement of foot and ankle disorders II: interclinician and intraclinician reliability and validity of the newly established standard rating scales and Japanese Orthopaedic Association rating scale. J Orthop Sci 2005; 10(5):466–74.
18. Albright R, Klein E, Baker J, et al. Are radiographs associated with patient satisfaction after scarf bunionectomy? J Foot Ankle Surg 2023;62(1):2–6.
19. Matthews M, Klein E, Youssef A, et al. Correlation of radiographic measurements with patient-centered outcomes in hallux valgus surgery. Foot Ankle Int 2018; 39(12):1416–22.

20. Srivastava S, Chockalingam N, El Fakhri T. Radiographic measurements of hallux angles: a review of current techniques. Foot 2010;20(1):27–31.
21. Srivastava S, Chockalingam N, El Fakhri T. Radiographic angles in hallux valgus: comparison between manual and computer-assisted measurements. J Foot Ankle Surg 2010;49(6):523–8.
22. Mattos EDMC, Freitas MF, Milano C, et al. Reliability of two smartphone applications for radiographic measurements of hallux valgus angles. J Foot Ankle Surg 2017;56(2):230–3.
23. Lin CS, Wu TY, Wang TM, et al. A new technique to increase reliability in measuring the axis of bone. J Foot Ankle Surg 2016;55(1):106–11.
24. Kuyucu E, Ceylan HH, Surucu S, et al. The effect of incorrect foot placement on the accuracy of radiographic measurements of the hallux valgus and inter-metatarsal angles for treating hallux valgus. Acta Chir Orthop Traumatol Cech 2017;84(3):196–201. Vliv nespravne polohy nohy na presnost radiologickeho mereni deformity a intermetatarzalnich uhlu pri leceni hallux valgus.
25. De Boer AS, Van Lieshout EMM, Vellekoop L, et al. The influence of radiograph obliquity on bohler's and gissane's angles in calcanei. J Foot Ankle Surg 2020; 59(1):44–7.
26. Banwell HA, Paris ME, Mackintosh S, et al. Paediatric flexible flat foot: how are we measuring it and are we getting it right? A systematic review. J Foot Ankle Res 2018;11:21.
27. Saltzman CL, Brandser EA, Berbaum KS, et al. Reliability of standard foot radiographic measurements. Foot Ankle Int 1994;15(12):661–5.
28. Kim Y, Kim JS, Young KW, et al. A new measure of tibial sesamoid position in hallux valgus in relation to the coronal rotation of the first metatarsal in CT scans. Foot Ankle Int 2015;36(8):944–52.
29. Dayton P, Feilmeier M, Kauwe M, et al. Relationship of frontal plane rotation of first metatarsal to proximal articular set angle and hallux alignment in patients under-going tarsometatarsal arthrodesis for hallux abducto valgus: a case series and critical review of the literature. J Foot Ankle Surg 2013;52(3):348–54.
30. Stacpoole-Shea S, Shea G, Otago L, et al. Instrumentation considerations of a clinical and a computerized technique for the measurement of foot angles. J Foot Ankle Surg 1998;37(5):410–5.
31. Rohan PY, Perrier A, Ramanoudjame M, et al. Three-dimensional reconstruction of foot in the weightbearing position from biplanar radiographs: evaluation of ac-curacy and reliability. J Foot Ankle Surg 2018;57(5):931–7.
32. de Cesar Netto C, Richter M. Use of advanced weightbearing imaging in evalu-ation of hallux valgus. Foot Ankle Clin 2020;25(1):31–45.
33. Heineman N, Xi Y, Zhang L, et al. Hallux valgus evaluation on MRI: can measure-ments validated on radiographs be used? J Foot Ankle Surg 2018;57(2):305–8.
34. Zhong Z, Zhang P, Duan H, et al. A comparison between X-ray imaging and an innovative computer-aided design method based on weightbearing CT scan im-ages for assessing hallux valgus. J Foot Ankle Surg 2021;60(1):6–10.
35. Gibboney MD, LaPorta GA, Dreyer MA. Interobserver analysis of standard foot and ankle radiographic angles. J Foot Ankle Surg 2019;58(6):1085–90.
36. Sheth S, Derner BS, Meyr AJ. Reliability of the measurement of cuboid height in midfoot charcot neuroarthropathy. J Foot Ankle Surg 2018;57(4):759–60.
37. Karthas TA, Cook JJ, Matthews MR, et al. Development and validation of the foot union scoring evaluation tool for arthrodesis of foot structures. J Foot Ankle Surg 2018;57(4):675–80.

38. Lawrence K, Doll H, McWhinnie D. Relationship between health status and post-operative return to work. J Public Health Med 1996;18(1):49–53.
39. Kitaoka HB, Meeker JE, Phisitkul P, et al. AOFAS position statement regarding patient-reported outcome measures. Foot Ankle Int 2018;39(12):1389–93.
40. Shibuya N, Kitterman RT, Jupiter DC. Evaluation of the rearfoot component (module 3) of the ACFAS scoring scale. J Foot Ankle Surg 2014;53(5):544–7.

Effective Case Reports and Small Case Series

Jason Piriano, DPM, MS[a,b], Thomas S. Roukis, DPM, PhD[a,b],*

KEYWORDS

- Education • Guideline • Publication • Research • Resident • Writing

KEY POINTS

- Case reports and small series play an important role in medical education because they permit detailed reporting of new pathology and unexpected effects as well as the study of causality.
- Case reports and small series have a high sensitivity for detecting novelty and provide many new concepts in patient care. As such, they remain a pillar of medical progress.
- Case reports and small series unfortunately have a lesser specificity for medical decision-making because by definition they lack homogeneity.
- Statistical analysis possibilities are limited, and generalization to a broader patient population should be avoided.
- Quality case reporting demands a clear focus to make explicit to the readers why a particular observation is important in the context of existing historical knowledge on the subject.

INTRODUCTION

Since the dawn of modern medicine, physicians have appreciated the intellectual stimulation afforded through the critical thinking obtained through detailed study of patient-specific problems.[1–5] Therefore, case reports and small series represent the ideal project for resident and fellow learners because the genesis of this form of research is less demanding than other forms of research to generate but still reinforce the discipline necessary to produce more complex and scientific research.[6] Coupled with the experience of a seasoned attending physician, case reports and small series provide the resident learner with the ability to display detective-like abilities and potentially ignite the motivation to explore an academic career.[7,8] However, without structure and a clear direction, great potential exists to over generalize the particulars of an isolated case report or small series of patients to the general population.[9] This

^a Department of Orthopaedics and Rehabilitation, University of Florida, College of Medicine-Jacksonville 655 West 8th Street, Jacksonville, FL, USA; ^b Residency Training-Podiatric Surgery, Department of Orthopaedics and Rehabilitation, University of Florida, College of Medicine-Jacksonville 655 West 8th Street, Jacksonville, FL, USA
* Corresponding author.
E-mail address: Thomas.Roukis@jax.ufl.edu

Clin Podiatr Med Surg 41 (2024) 269–272
https://doi.org/10.1016/j.cpm.2023.08.001
0891-8422/24/© 2023 Elsevier Inc. All rights reserved.

podiatric.theclinics.com

would potentially expose patients to harm and as such case reports and small series should be reviewed carefully.

RESEARCH TRIANGLE
What Makes an Effective Case Report? What Is "Unique"?

Case reports and small series exist to highlight novel or unique therapeutic approaches or variations on a multitude of factors involved with patient care. It may be the unexpected outcome from a surgical technique, the excellent outcomes with fixation constructs, or adverse outcome that begin to pave the way for what future studies should focus on. It may even highlight an important complication seldom overlooked, minimally discussed, or rarely reported. Bottom line, an effective case report is one that begins to turn the cogwheels within the readers head on the subject being evaluated, is portrayed as a captivating story that weaves narratives and context for the readers while delivering content about the patient's journey—with all relevant history of present illness, imaging, laboratory results, and follow-up documented. The interpretation that the reader takes away from the novel or rare presentation is what makes case reports so integral within the scientific field. This, in essence, is what makes each case report and small series so unique.[10,11]

What Does an Effective Literature Review for a Case Report Look Like? How Many References Should Be Cited? How Much Detail Reported?

The foundation of a great case report and small series stems from its literature review. The context of one's case report must be seen through the lens of existing literature and knowledge. It is this foundation that reinforces the claims made, the rationale for the case report itself, and most importantly, the evidence to support the research itself. The number of references varies depending on the topic at hand. Generally, 10 to 20 references would be an acceptable range that covers the diversity of the subject, the existing knowledge briefly, and would not be overwhelming to the article. The number of references should be limited to either greater than 5 or less than 30 as the focus should be to select the most contemporary literature with enough background information to compare and contrast one's claim(s). The detail needs to be terse and to the point; extrapolating what is critically necessary within a few sentences, a paragraph at most, for adequate comprehensive dialogue within the discussion section.[10,11]

What Information Is Valuable to Include in a Case Report? What Is Superfluous?

Information presented in case reports and small series should be informative, specific, and relevant. How one defines relevancy depends on the focus of case report/series. In addition, it should assist in answering questions or stirring dialogue about the topic at hand. The author's goal is to extrapolate data or statements that would either support their claims or refute others. Regardless of the intention, the focus must be based on the evidence. Whether it is a complication or an outcome, the data must be available to support the claim. Ultimately, justifiable evidence-based conclusions are the essence of valuable information within the construct of the ones case report/series. Anything besides that would be considered superfluous.[11–13]

Case Report Versus Case Series

Case reports add significant value as they relate to novel techniques and methods, diagnosis, and procedures as well as aid in establishing a proof of concept. Case reports drive progress and furthermore could be viewed from the perspective that it lays the foundation for a case series. From a scientific and statistical perspective, multiple replicates are crucial to quantify and establish evidence. Per definition, a small case series is a series of multiple case reports, in which said individuals have similar characteristics and have received similar treatment and can therefore be compared side by side. It is an accurate representation of a pattern of outcomes that can be used for novel discovery and/or to prove or reject a hypothesis. The level of evidence associated with either plays a minimal role as both case series and studies are level 4 evidence.[10–13]

Tips and Techniques for Pictures/Figures/Tables

The most important critical aspect of any manuscript, albeit retrospective studies or randomized clinical trials, is the presentation of data itself. Figures and tables must include relevant data that stands out and captures the attention of the reader, that is, clean, easy to read/follow and makes coherent sense. Certain color contrast panels or fonts may assist in drawing attention or improving readability, but the foundation lies with the choice of presentation (bar graphs, innovating diagrams, tables, and so forth). When pictures are submitted, assisting the reader with labels, arrows or circles superimposed onto images can be quite helpful, especially with images of anatomy. Readers tend to focus on the discussion and data itself, so having these principles adhered to can significantly improve one's work. The quantity of imaging per submission should be confirmed by the allotted amount per submission by the journal you wish to submit to. Limitations aside, three to five pictures, figures, tables would be an acceptable range for any submission within case reports and series.[10–13]

WHAT CONCLUSIONS CAN BE DRAWN FOR CASE REPORTS? WHAT CONCLUSIONS EXTRAPOLATE TOO MUCH?

Case reports have one specific goal in mind when submitted: trends. Their purpose is to advance anecdotal evidence or professional opinion into trends that seem factual and are not by coincidence. With multiple case reports, case series begin to rise ultimately leading to cohort studies, pilot studies, and comparative studies, which lead to systematic reviews and meta-analysis. They contribute to the advancement of literature and evidence-based medicine overtime. Although very integral to how medicine functions, one must be careful as to the interpretation of the data. Case reports are not the gospel and must be interpreted with caution as multiple types of bias exist in the literature and must be taken into consideration.[14] Case reports are not designed to make powerful statements such as meta-analyses and systematic reviews are able to, but to simply advise on trends or tendencies associated with the topic at hand which may or may not be by coincidence. With case reports and case series, the frame of mind of the reader and author must be in accordance with associated level of evidence. Only then, can the conclusions drawn from literature, the evidence-based medicine itself, be applied to the fullest.

CLINICS CARE POINTS

- Case reports and series represent the time-honored approach to patient-centric care.
- Case reports and series have the potential for multiple forms of bias.
- Case reports and series should be seen as supplementing higher level of evidence scientific studies as they are not generalizable to larger patient populations.
- Statistical analysis possibilities are limited and generalization to a broader patient population should be avoided.

CONFLICTS OF INTEREST

The authors have nothing to disclose.

REFERENCES

1. Nayak BK. The significance of case reports in biomedical publication. Indian J Ophthalmol 2010;58(5):363.
2. Borracci RA. The value of publishing case reports in the era of evidence-based medicine. Rev Argent Cardiol 2016;84(6):568–9.
3. Thorne JE. Weighing the evidence: evaluating contributions from case reports and case series. Retin Cases Brief Rep 2012;6(4):337–8.
4. Twa MD. The value of clinical case reports in evidence-based practice. Optom Vis Sci 2017;94(2):135–6.
5. Packer CD, Katz RB, Iacopetti CL, et al. A case suspended in time: the educational value of case reports. Acad Med 2017;92(2):152–6.
6. Ortega-Loubon C, Culquichicón C, Correa R. The importance of writing and publishing case reports during medical training. Cureus 2017;9(12):e1964.
7. Florek AG, Dellavalle RP. Case reports in medical education: a platform for training medical students, residents, and fellows in scientific writing and critical thinking. J Med Case Rep 2016;10:1–3.
8. Merchant A, Chastain P. Role of case reports in modern medical education. Clin Case Rep Rv 2018;4(6):2.
9. Karami H, Rezapour M, Naderisorki M. Writing a case report correctly; from edwin smith papyrus to the CARE statement. Clinical Excellence 2021;10(4):33–40.
10. Grapsa J. How to write your first clinical case report. Case Reports 2022;4(21):1456–8.
11. Nield LS. Writing case reports for the clinical literature: practical approach for the novice author. Journal of Graduate Medical Education 2011;3(3):445.
12. Juyal D, Thaledi S, Thawani V. Writing patient case reports for publication. Educ Health 2013;26(2):126–9.
13. Heller M, Kontzialis M, Anderson A, et al. From the editor's desk: common errors in submission of case reports. Radiology Case Reports 2012;7(4):771.
14. Roukis TS. Case reports/series & bias considerations. Foot Ankle Surg: Techniques, Reports & Cases 2021;1(3). https://doi.org/10.1016/j.fastrc.2021.100057.

Critical Analysis of Retrospective Study Designs
Cohort and Case Series

Emily Lobos, DPM[a], Alan Catanzariti, DPM[b],*, Ryan McMillen, DPM[b]

KEYWORDS

- Retrospective study • Cohort study • Case series

KEY POINTS

- To interpret retrospective studies, one must understand their inherent limitations as well as critically analyze the methods, results, and discussion sections of a paper to determine its validity and possible application to clinical practice.
- Designing a retrospective study has its relative advantages and disadvantages as well as special considerations. Limitations must be unabashedly acknowledged in the discussion to help readers better interpret results and apply the conclusions that are reached.
- Retrospective cohort studies examine larger groups of patients with a similar outcome or exposure and are either compared with a matched group or examined alone. Case series follow small groups of patients, all with similar outcomes or exposure. Both are beneficial for studying variables for which one might not easily or ethically investigate with a randomized control trial methodology.

INTRODUCTION

Retrospective studies are one of the most popular research study designs. This can be attributed to the availability of data, ease of data collection, and lower overall cost. However, there is the presumption that the quality of data presented in retrospective studies is inferior to that of prospective methodologies. One might argue that this is not a fair assessment of this type of research, especially in the context of the niche in which it is most beneficial.

Case series are retrospective reviews of small groups of patients, usually defined as greater than four but less than twenty, which share the same unique exposure or outcome. These studies are best used for rare diseases or outcomes in which a larger

[a] Department of Orthopedics, Division of Foot and Ankle Surgery, West Penn Hospital, 4800 Friendship Avenue, N1, Pittsburgh, PA 15224, USA; [b] Department of Orthopedics, West Penn Hospital Foot & Ankle Surgery, Allegheny Health Network, 4800 Friendship Avenue, N1, Pittsburgh, PA 15224, USA
* Corresponding author. West Penn Hospital, Foot and Ankle institute, 4800 Friendship Avenue, N1, Pittsburgh, PA 15224.
E-mail address: alan.catanzariti@ahn.org

Clin Podiatr Med Surg 41 (2024) 273–280
https://doi.org/10.1016/j.cpm.2023.09.002
0891-8422/24/© 2023 Elsevier Inc. All rights reserved.

podiatric.theclinics.com

group for study could not be collected, but the study of their common exposure or outcome could be beneficial to current patients or serve as an inspiration to other scientists for larger projects on the matter. Although data from these studies are descriptive in nature, it can still be compelling and helpful to clinicians.

Retrospective cohort studies examine a larger group of participants and usually are structured in one of two ways. In the first, the group has a common exposure, and researchers are identifying intermediate or long-term outcomes that the group has in common. In the second, they identify a group with a common outcome and retrospectively examine their medical and social history to find possible common exposures. In either instance, retrospective cohort studies are effective at examining research questions that would be unethical or not feasible to perform as prospective studies. For example, retrospective cohort studies of lung cancer found that smoking cigarettes was a common exposure and likely a main contributor. It would be unethical to create a prospective study based on this question as intentionally exposing someone to smoking, a harmful exposure, would be unethical. Retrospective studies have several strengths and weaknesses. It is important to understand a retrospective study's purpose, how to critically examine them, and how to design them for clinicians to know when they are applicable to their practice.

RETROSPECTIVE DESIGN OVERVIEW

Retrospective studies are incredibly common in podiatric literature for several reasons. As might be expected, there are advantages and disadvantages to this form of research. Beginning with the advantages, one of the greatest is that retrospective studies generally produce results quickly and with meager costs.[1] A retrospective study does not require recruitment of patients, significant time spent waiting for results postexposure, or time collecting data points such as surveys or reaching out to patients over the phone. For some retrospective studies, a researcher only needs to find and contact a patient once for updated information versus following them over many years.[1] For other studies, the patients do not even need to be contacted at all and all data points can be collected from chart review as soon as the study is approved by an institutional review board. Put simply, unlike prospective or interventional studies, retrospective studies have already completed the long interval of time between exposure and outcome, making data collection generally quick and easy.[1] Another advantage is the comprehensive nature of cohort studies. Interventional or prospective studies are often focused on a single primary outcome, whereas a cohort study might determine the natural history of exposure and the spectrum of outcomes following it.[1]

Arguably the greatest advantage of a retrospective study design is the ability to study elements that would be ethically impossible to incorporate into a randomized control trial (RCT). Smoking is an example of a beneficial retrospective study that could never be an RCT.[2] One cannot ethically place patients in a randomized group that exposes them to an element that is known to be or strongly believed to be harmful. However, it is still critical that these elements be studied. This is where retrospective designs thrive.

The limitations of retrospective studies are numerous but unavoidable. First, a temporal sequence of events—exposure followed by outcome—does not ensure or imply a causal relationship.[1] This is how data are collected in retrospective studies and it is easy to misinterpret this direction of events to be meaningful when they are not, in fact, linked. Furthermore, data for retrospective studies are not collected in a predesigned systematic way. Therefore, some data will inevitably be missing or recorded in a form that does not align with the collection format desired by the researcher. In addition, there could be variables that affect the outcome the researcher is searching for that may not have been recorded at all. These issues create unknown or unnoticed biases in the data.[2] When those certain variables are missing, researchers might ask the patient to recall these events and place them in time or analyze surrounding notes for estimates of the exposure and/or outcome timing. This might also cause bias secondary to fallacious patient recall or estimates within note taking that is not explicitly stated.[2]

The most important limitation of an observational retrospective study is the lack of randomization. The patients' exposure is not randomized. Instead, it is chosen by the participant or physician based on participant characteristics. For example, in a retrospective study comparing those in a cohort who received treatment for their ailment and those who did not, the patients receiving the treatment are more likely to be at a higher disease level because the physician determined intervention was the appropriate route.[1] This can create confounding variables that make it difficult for the researcher and reader to parse out what is an important contributing factor to the outcome, and what is not connected.

This is commonly known as a selection bias. Using a podiatric example, if a retrospective study was designed to investigate the difference in outcomes between a triple versus double rearfoot arthrodesis, it is effectively impossible to determine why the surgeon initially determined to recommend a double versus triple arthrodesis to each specific patient. There must have been some reason why one procedure was recommended versus the other, but it is unfeasible to determine what that reason was in retrospect. Prospective randomization removes this uncertainly and selection bias.

CASE SERIES VERSUS COHORT

It is important to understand the levels of evidence when reviewing and digesting research material. Level I evidence includes randomized controlled trials that show a significant difference between treatment groups or achieve a narrow confidence interval. Level II includes both RCTs with less than 80% follow-up rate and prospective cohort studies. Level III includes retrospective cohort studies and case-control studies. Level IV includes retrospective case series.[3] With these outlined, we can place retrospective studies in Levels III and IV. Because Levels I and II are prospective in nature, retrospective design studies effectively cannot ever fall into these categories.

A case series can be defined as multiple, similar instructive cases that might be used to study rare and unusual diseases. Case series normally involve one group of patients. In these studies, follow-up is inconsistent and there are no controls. The likelihood of bias in these studies is high, secondary to researchers' selection of cases that are all linked to an outcome of interest. Another definition of a case series is a "descriptive retrospective study," meaning that most of the data are qualitative rather than quantitative.[3] Case descriptions can be beneficial in helping others generate hypotheses for future research and study designs.[2]

Subject cohorts must be carefully defined in the setting of research studies. One definition of cohort is a collection or group, usually of the same demographics. For example, people of the same age while in school are often called a cohort. However, in research, a cohort study is more specific and involves groups of subjects that researchers study over time, looking for the development of a disease or outcome after a specific and shared exposure.[3] The patients are either all in a single cohort that shares the exposure, or there are two separate groups split into those who experienced exposure and those that did not. In either case, the members of a cohort should share as many similarities as possible to mitigate possible confounding variables.

INTERPRETING RESEARCH

A physician must be able to interpret research even if they do not plan to conduct it. The methods, results, and discussion sections must be closely examined to understand if the research and its outcomes are relevant to one's practice. Bhandari and colleagues suggest a three-step approach to interpreting research and letting it aid in patient care. First, assess whether the study can provide valid results. In other words, does the study have internal validity? Second, review the results in full. And third, consider how the results might be applied to your patients, or how generalizable these results are.[4]

In an overview, the *methods* section should describe what was done to analyze the research question proposed within the introduction, describe the steps taken to complete this, and justify the experimental design.[5] The methods section includes the information by which the study's validity can be judged. It should be structured in a way that the reader is able to determine both internal and external validity of the study. Internal validity describes the credibility of the study and whether the conclusions drawn correctly describe what actually transpired during the study. The external validity refers to what degree the results of a study can be generalized to a more global population.[5] Judging external validity can be aided by two things within the methods section: first, the descriptive data regarding basic demographics of the cohort—this is normally included in Table 1 of the paper. These statistics include age, gender, comorbidities, and other data relevant in the context of the study. The second is analyzing who was chosen for inclusion in the study. This will determine what limits are placed on how far the generalization can be stretched.[5]

The concept of "Table 1" is an extremely important concept when considering the interpretation and application of results from retrospective study designs. The study investigators should attempt to provide as much descriptive data as possible in order to adequately define their study cohort. Subsequently, a critical reader should individually assess the patient characteristics described in Table 1 and make an independent assessment about whether or not these characteristics are similar to patients they see in their own practice. For example, patients with midfoot Charcot neuroarthropathy in urban Pittsburgh, Pennsylvania, are likely to share some, but not all, of the characteristics of patients with midfoot Charcot neuroarthropathy in rural Australia. Therefore, an investigation into midfoot Charcot neuroarthropathy patients from Pittsburgh might have some, but likely not complete applicability to Australian physicians. It depends on the critical reader and not the study investigators, to determine whether or not results are applicable.

More specifically, there are key points within this section that should be noted by the critical reader. In a case series, an important point is the inclusion criteria for the patients within the series. In a cohort study, one should examine the demographic description of the cohorts being compared and recognize how similar or dissimilar they are. Another important point is the duration of follow-up for the patients in both types of studies. This will allow for clarification on the time elapsed between exposure and outcome. It should also be clear to the reader after analyzing the methods section in its totality why a retrospective design was chosen.

To distill it down, the scientific approach to research is based on a controlled and critical examination of an issue. Statistics are the tool that allows us to communicate how likely the results of this approach were to have occurred by chance.[6] The *results* portion of a research paper can often be overwhelming if one is not familiar with the associated statistical tests. However, there are a few key points that might be used to determine the paper's validity and understand the authors' conclusions. First, one should pay attention to the choice of statistics used by the authors. This will be dependent on the nature of what is being measured and should match the type of data the authors put forth as being collected in the methods section.[6] Descriptive statistics are simply those used to describe the characteristics of a group, for example, the group's age, gender, comorbidities, and so forth. These statistics are not meant to be generalized to other groups and are meant to give the reader an overview of the type of patient being studied.[6] The ability to generalize to other groups requires inferential statistics. These are used to allow the reader to attempt to predict the behavior of a large group based on the experience with the small group that is the research subject at hand. Examples include t-tests, analysis of variance (ANOVAS), chi squares, and others. These will have associated probability values (P values), which are used to help the reader determine if the statistical is significant. By definition, statistical significance is an estimate of the probability that an outcome inference or generalization is genuine. These P values are used in research because one can never be absolutely sure that the effect can be generalized to the larger population from the representative sample size. This value does not represent a measure or magnitude of an effect.[6] A significant P value is known to be 0.05 or less in scientific literature. This means that the possibility that an effect happened at random is 5%, or 1 in 20. In plain speak, this means to consider an effect statistically significant, it must be more than likely the difference is due to the treatment and not to chance or variation.[6]

Noting the P value is an important step. However, one must also differentiate between statistical and clinical significance of an outcome within a research study. Statistical significance reflects the likelihood that this outcome is generalizable to the larger population. Clinical significance reflects the clinical value of an outcome, or whether the changes were large enough to make the treatment worthwhile to the clinician.[6] Confidence intervals are a useful tool in determining the clinical significance of an outcome. Confidence intervals offer a better indication of the strength of the inference that one can draw from the data than P values alone. They are given in the same units as the results being assessed, in turn indicating that the limits within which the difference between two and more treatments are likely to be found. The most common is a 95% confidence interval. This is the range of values that a researcher is 95% certain that includes the mean of the population as a whole. As a sample size increases, the confidence interval decreases. The researcher can be more confident that a tighter range includes the population generalizable value.[6]

A close reading of both the methods and results of any retrospective study will inevitably demonstrate confounding variables. These are variables that are not manipulated by the investigator and are also not the main focus of the study, but still have the ability to affect the relationships between predictors and outcome. In other words, any extraneous variable may affect the dependent variable that is not the independent variable of interest.[5] These can sometimes cause a false appearance of reversal of results.[1] Examples of confounding factors that often occur include disease or injury severity, race, or socioeconomic status.[1] Researchers cannot avoid these altogether, but authors should attempt to mitigate these or acknowledge them within the discussion section. If there are obvious confounding variables not recognized within the paper, the reader is responsible for recognizing these themselves.

When assessing the research paper results sections, keep in mind the statistics that make general sense to run in the setting of the methods and hypothesis of the specific paper. If the data are not presented with straightforward statistics, there could be ulterior motives at play. A few possibilities include weak trends that influence the author to obscure these with unusual statistical tests, bias toward the result presented by certain tests even if they are not appropriate in the setting, or the author having a limited knowledge of statistical test therefore applying only the ones they know even if they are out of context.[6]

The *discussion* section gives the reader a chance to understand how the authors interpret their results along with the literature they use to support these interpretations. Using the aforementioned strategies for interpreting the data should allow for the ability to critically read the discussion section. A thorough analysis of the discussion section should either confirm or debunk the clinical relevance of the paper that one should have determined based on the methods and results sections.

However, one of the most important subsections of the discussion should be placed near the end of the paper: acknowledgment of the limitations of the study. Limitations are inherent to all study methodologies. Authors should be honest with their limitations and recognize any issues with the sample—whether bias or size, any unmitigated confounding variables, short follow-up times, or other issues. If an author does not have a thorough limitations section, the reader should be even more critical of the piece as a whole. Limitations do not speak to failures of the authors in their methodological design. Instead they represent the prism in which the results of an investigation should be viewed. Therefore, the limitations portion of an investigation should represent an honest and open discussion about the relative restraints of a methodology and not simply a required listing of potential flaws. This represents a chance for the authors to speak to readers about how results might be best interpreted.

As the reader, you must be the final quality control filter on a research paper. A retrospective study that has been published does not intrinsically equate to a quality study or manuscript. Before allowing a paper to influence your practice, you must thoroughly vet the quality of the research using the tools outlined above.[6] Some common pitfalls in statistics should be on your radar during a critical reading of the research literature. Watch for those who use statistical significance to suggest a clinical effect. Look out for those who use statistical methods that do not fit their methods or the context. These studies should be scrutinized to find the reason why they are using a relatively obscure approach. Always read a paper with the statistical power of the sample in mind. This is important in determining whether generalizations can be made from a certain study. If a paper states that there is no difference between two groups without adequate statistical power within the sample, this is false. It is possible that there is a difference, but the sample size used was too small to detect this. It would better be reported in that case as "inconclusive."[6]

An important step in becoming a consumer of research is the development of skills needed to critically evaluate the research. Although the journal in which the study is contained can give some indication of its merit, it cannot be used entirely to judge the validity of the study.[7] Generally, one must evaluate research critically before allowing the findings to influence their clinical judgment.

Some important criteria to evaluate on include: are the theories supported by valid anatomic and physiologic evidence? Does their literature review include peer-reviewed studies that support their research question and possibly theory? Are limitations of the study discussed candidly? Are potential side effects or complications of the treatment discussed presented? And is the conclusion made for a specific population?[7]

DESIGNING A STUDY

Three important factors should help guide your research method decision-making. First, evidence: understanding the outcomes you are hoping to elucidate and which method would best help you achieve this. Next, the subject and researcher factors:

the individual needs of a population, the researchers' previous experiences, and accounting for participant limitations. Finally, constraints: the cost of the study, availability of equipment, time availability of the subjects, and researcher.[8] Common stages include: identifying a question to be explored, identifying a population in which to test for an effect, selecting an appropriate sample, recording the exposure, and collecting data points after exposure that are related to the effect you are studying.[8] Retrospective studies are chosen to collect information about a sample population in regard to the occurrence of a specific outcome or phenomenon that has already taken place. Like stated before, this type of study has advantages and disadvantages that one must take into consideration. Retrospective research, like all other clinical research designs, requires a clinical question that can be answered scientifically. Therefore, the question must be closed-ended with defined interrelated variables, usually referred to as the independent and dependent variable, and able to be measured in a way that is amenable to statistical analysis.[9] More specifically, a research question best answered by retrospective design is one of two things. It is either a question that can be answered by a population who has already undergone the exposure and a period of time postexposure in which you can look at outcomes. Alternatively, it is a question that can be answered by a population who has the outcome you would like to study and you can retrospectively review their history to find common exposures within the cohort.

Once you have a question appropriate for retrospective design, you must decide how to structure your methods. First, you must make decisions on your sample size. Because this is not prospective, it is not amenable to simply picking how many people you would like to enroll. Begin your query with broad inclusion criteria for either the population with the exposure or outcome you would like to interrogate. Based on the number of possible participants returned from this query, you can narrow your inclusion criteria until either it is as narrow as you desire, or the population is too small to have statistical power. Another consideration that will impact the size of the cohort is the length of follow-up postexposure. Logically, longer longitudinal follow time is better; however, you must weigh this against the data available for your cohort and the rate of attrition. There is no minimum or maximum follow-up time. An ideal time is one that is as long as possible while still obtaining an answer to your research question and keeping a cohort with a population size large enough to be statistically powerful. Finally, when designing a retrospective study, particularly a cohort design, one must avoid confounding variables by trying to match the subjects within each cohort by their age, gender, comorbidities, and so forth. When writing the methods section within a manuscript, it is important to describe materials used in the execution of the study, an explanation of how measurements were made, the statistical tests and calculations that were performed in the analysis of the data, and justification for the experimental design.[5] The methods section must be written in a way that is clear and logical so that the experiment could be reproduced by others to evaluate the results as well as allowing the reader to judge whether the results and conclusions are valid.[5]

When performing a retrospective case series, the data will be qualitative. Therefore, there are no statistical tests to run. Often, the data are reported as how many of the patients in the case series had certain traits before exposure and then the varied outcomes postexposure. In cohort studies, the results section should include the statistical findings when carrying out the tests and calculations described within the methods section. This normally includes t-tests, ANOVAS, P values, confidence intervals, and varied others depending on the type of data being reviewed and the size of the cohort. P values and confidence intervals were described in the previous headed section. The commonality between the two types of retrospective studies is the importance of a thorough Table 1. Within an article, Table 1 should contain a summary of the important demographics of either each member of a case series or the statistical representation of demographics among the members of a cohort study. This allows a reader to view a sort of summary of the population you are reviewing. By being contained within the first table of the paper, readers can quickly know where to reference this information.

The discussion section should discuss the findings of the study in the context of other similar literature and their findings. The most important aspect for a retrospective study will be acknowledging the study's limitations. For retrospective studies, this is often the sample size, the length of follow-up time, data collection modality, and possible confounding variables. It is important to note that retrospective studies are known to either underestimate or overestimate the treatment effects.[4] A paper's author should be candid about any limitations in order to help the reader better contextualize the paper as a whole and decide whether it is of clinical value to them.

Retrospective case series and cohort studies are valuable tools for those consuming research and those creating it. Better understanding how they are created and how to interpret them will assist in the consumption and application of research to clinical practice. Every research style has an important place within the greater field of scientific research.

DISCLOSURE

The authors have no financial disclosures.

REFERENCES

1. Parker RA, Berman NG. Cohort studies. In: Parker RA, Berman NG, editors. *Planning critical research*. 1st edition. Cambridge, MA, USA: Cambridge University Press; 2016. p. 82–94.
2. Talari K, Goyal M. Retrospective studies - utility and caveats. J Roy Coll Phys Edinb 2020;50(4):398–402.
3. Poehling GG, Jenkins CB. Levels of evidence and your therapeutic study: what's the difference with cohorts, controls and cases? Arthrosc J Arthrosc Relat Surg 2004;20(6):563.
4. Bhandari M, Guyatt GH, Swiontkowski MF. User's guide to the orthopaedic literature: how to use an article about a surgical therapy. J Bone Joint Surg 2001; 83-A(6):916–26.
5. Kallet RH. How to write the methods section of a research paper. Respir Care 2004;49(10):1229–32.
6. Redmond AC, Keenan AM. Understanding statistics: Putting p-values into perspective. J Am Podiatr Med Assoc 2002;92(5):297–305.
7. Keenan AM, Redmond AC. Integrating research into the clinic: what evidence based practice means to the practising podiatrist. J Am Podiatr Med Assoc 2002;92(2):115–22.
8. Redmond AC, Keenan AM, Landorf K. 'Horses for courses': the differences between quantitative and qualitative approaches to research. J Am Podiatr Med Assoc 2002;92(3):159–69.
9. Hendrix P, Griessenauer C. Retrospective analysis from a chart review: a step-by-step guide. In: Shoja MM, et al, editors. *A guide to the scientific career: Virtues, communication, research, and Academic writing*. 1st edition. Hoboken, NJ, USA: John Wiley & Sons, Inc; 2020. p. 263–6.

Prospective Surgical Cohort Analysis

Adam E. Fleischer, DPM, MPH[a,b,c,*], Rachel H. Albright, DPM, MPH[d,1]

KEYWORDS

- Appraisal • Evidence-based medicine • Chance • Bias • Confounding
- Journal club • Podiatry • Foot

KEY POINTS

- We recommend a 3-step approach when critically appraising a prospective surgical cohort study, which involves examining the study's *generalizability*, *results*, and finally its overall *validity*.
- When determining generalizability, look at the patient demographics, inclusion/exclusion criteria, and description of the surgical technique and surgeon(s) skill level, and determine whether the study findings may be applicable to your practice and patient population.
- When examining the *results*, ask 2 questions: (1) How *large* was the treatment effect and (2) How *precise* was the estimate of the treatment effect? Precision will tell you how likely it is that *chance* might have influenced the study findings.
- Assessing a study's *validity* should include a systematic evaluation of the possible *biases* and uncontrolled *confounders*. When randomization is used to assign group allocation, and it is successful, the threat of confounding is severely minimized.

INTRODUCTION

Prospective enrollment of subjects allows for the opportunity to significantly minimize many of the biases (eg, selection, nonresponder, and interviewer) that often plague less tightly controlled retrospective foot/ankle studies. Prospective cohort studies are inherently more rigorous than their retrospective counterparts, both in their conduct and in design, as they require participant consent and must pass the rigors of Institutional Review Board *approval* (not merely exemption) before being initiated. As such,

a Podiatric Medicine & Surgery Residency Program, Advocate Illinois Masonic Medical Center/RFUMS, Chicago, IL, USA; b Weil Foot & Ankle Institute, Chicago, IL, USA; c Department of Podiatric Medicine & Surgery, Rosalind Franklin University of Medicine & Science (RFUMS), 3333 Green Bay Road, North Chicago, IL 60064, USA; d Foot & Ankle Surgery, Department of Surgery, Stamford Health Medical Group, Stamford, CT, USA
1 Present address: 800 Post Road, Suite 302, Darien, CT 06820.
* Corresponding author. Department of Podiatric Medicine & Surgery, Rosalind Franklin University of Medicine & Science (RFUMS), 3333 Green Bay Road, North Chicago, IL 60064.
E-mail address: adam.e.fleischer@gmail.com

Clin Podiatr Med Surg 41 (2024) 281–290
https://doi.org/10.1016/j.cpm.2023.07.005
0891-8422/24/© 2023 Elsevier Inc. All rights reserved.
podiatric.theclinics.com

we assign a high(er) level of evidence to the conclusions reached in cohort studies with a prospective design.

A cohort is a group of patients, ideally at a similar place in their disease progression, exposed to one or more interventions and followed forward until they reach an outcome. Exposure (or treatment) allocation is determined randomly (eg, via the flip of a coin) in clinical level of evidence (CLOE) 1 and 2 cohort studies. These are commonly referred to as randomized controlled trails (RCTs). Therapeutic CLOE 3 studies also have a treatment and control (or comparison) group but differ in that group allocation is instead *non*randomized. Randomization is important because it diminishes the potential for confounders (both known and those yet unknown) to interfere with the interpretation of the study's results. When random group assignments are not performed, investigators must go to great lengths using either a matched study design or highly sophisticated multivariable analyses to account for the effects of potential confounders. Because these methods are never perfect at eliminating the threat of confounding, many academicians contend that therapeutic articles that are CLOE 3 (and below) can be no better than "hypothesis generating" in their conclusions. With that said, rigorous RCTs comparing foot/ankle surgical therapies continue to be a rarity in the United States. Therefore, as surgeons and consumers of scientific literature, we should possess the basic skills needed to critically appraise both randomized and nonrandomized prospective cohort study designs.

It is our intention with this article that it might serve as an abbreviated "user's guide" for attending surgeons, residents and fellow trainees, and students when critiquing prospective surgical cohort studies. It is based loosely off a similar review published by Bhandari and colleagues,[1] and it follows closely much of the published material on critically appraising therapeutic studies accessible on Oxford's Centre for Evidence Based Medicine website.[2] We chose to limit the scope of the article to include only cohort studies with a comparison group (ie, CLOE 3 and above) because these provide us with the greatest value when making clinical and surgical decisions. We also illustrate this process in the context of preparing for and conducting a journal club session with your peers, house staff, and so forth.

SELECTING AND CRITIQUING AN ARTICLE IS A 3-STEP PROCESS

When deciding which articles to include in journal club sessions at our hospital, we ask ourselves 2 questions even *before* selecting the article for full review and *before* doing a deep dive into the article's validity: (1) How generalizable/applicable will these findings be to *our* patients (Step 1) and (2) How meaningful are the findings/study results (Step 2)?

In a quick 10-to-15-minute survey of potential articles, we ask, Can these results be applied to my patients? In other words, if I accept everything that the authors conclude, can I start applying the information tomorrow? If the answer is "no" because the patient population, or surgeon's technique/skill level, and so forth is too dissimilar from our own, then it is usually not an article that we entertain and dissect any further. This is generally referred to as the study's applicability or generalizability and can readily be found by examining the patient demographics (typically found in **Table 1**). The patient population and problem being studied (the P, in P-I-C-O) is also further defined in the methods section as the inclusion and exclusion criteria are further detailed. Surgeon abilities and operative technique(s) (the I and C, in P-I-C-O) can also be readily ascertained from the methods section.

The next thing we will focus on during our initial review of potential articles is the study results (the O, in P-I-C-O). This sounds simple, yet most trainees and

Table 1
Measures (in boldface) used to quantify the *magnitude of the treatment effect*

Treatment Group (Midfoot Fusion + STJ Fusion)		Control Group (Midfoot Fusion Alone)					
No. of events/No. of surgeries	Rate of progression (X) (%)	No. of events/No. of surgeries	Rate of progression (Y) (%)	Absolute Risk Reduction (ARR) (%)	Relative Risk (RR)	Relative Risk Reduction (RRR)	No. of patients needed to treat (NNT)
8/28	28.5	14/44	31.8	3.3	0.896	0.104	30

Event, progression onto ankle Charcot neuroarthropathy. ARR, risk of the outcome in the control group (Y) – risk of the outcome in the treatment group (X). This is also known as the absolute risk difference. RR, risk of the outcome in the treatment group/risk of the outcome in the control group, or 0.285/0.318 or 0.033 or 3.3%. RRR, absolute risk reduction/risk of the outcome in the control group. An alternative way to calculate the RRR is to subtract the RR from 1 (eg, RRR = 1–RR), or 1 – 0.896, or 0.104 or 10.4%. NNT, inverse of the ARR and is calculated as 1/ARR, or 1/0.033, or 30.

practitioners will read the results of published articles and recite them word for word when articulating the study's findings to others. However, it is not always the case that the authors stated results mirror the study's actual results. In fact, it is quite rare to see an author put their findings into such great perspective that further thought/deliberation is not needed. The results section, rather, requires serious contemplation. I recommend this reflection be done *early* when deciding whether the article is worthy of your focus during a journal club with others. When examining the authors' results, the 2 primary questions to ask are as follows: (1) How *large* was the treatment effect and (2) How *precise* was the estimate of the treatment effect? If the treatment effect is small despite statistical significance being reported in the article, the article is probably not going to change the way one treats the problem/ patient (P) or condition. Furthermore, if the treatment effect is large but the precision of the estimate is wide-ranging, and ranges from potentially negligible (no effect) to substantial, then that too requires further investigation and is unlikely to change the way one practices.

Once you have found a comparative article using a similar patient population/problem as your own, with familiar surgeons/operative techniques, reporting sufficiently large treatment effects with some level of precision, this then has the potential to change the way you treat your patients starting tomorrow. You have now found an article that is worthy of a journal club session. At our hospital, journal club sessions serve as an opportunity to critically appraise the validity (Step 3) of the authors' reported findings in an open forum. Most articles we come across will not pass the first and second steps of both being generally applicable to our population and contain results that could meaningfully change the way in which we treat our patients. However, once that bar has been passed, the real excitement begins! Below, we describe the 3 distinct appraisal steps in greater detail.

STEP 1: APPLICABILITY/GENERALIZABILITY OF THE STUDY'S FINDINGS
Can the Results Be Applied to My Patients?

I recommend asking this first, before getting too deep "in the weeds." I remember, several years ago, participating in a collaborative journal club session between our hospital's department of vascular surgery and podiatry section. We were interested in examining whether patients with diabetes and foot ulcers and severe peripheral lower extremity arterial disease ([P], Population) would be better served with open arterial bypass surgery ([I], Intervention) or percutaneous angioplasty ([C], Comparator). At that time, a large multicenter study conducted in the United Kingdom had just been published, entitled "The Bypass versus Angioplasty in Severe Ischemia of the Leg (BASIL) trial."[3] This was at the time, and remains to this day, the only randomized controlled trial comparing open surgical bypass with endovascular therapy for limb ischemia. It was not until 30 minutes into our rather rigorous appraisal of the article that it became clear this study would not help us answer our question (P-I-C-O). We were looking for the best option for *our* patients with *diabetes* and peripheral arterial disease, which typically involves multisegmented arterial occlusions distal to the knee, whereas the BASIL trial population consisted predominantly of nondiabetic patients (58% of the 452 subjects) with proximal lower extremity arterial occlusions. In fact, most bypass procedures and angioplasties were performed from the femoral to popliteal arteries, with relatively few reaching to the distal tibial or peroneal arteries of the leg. We realized, only after considerable effort, that the applicability and generalizability, then, of the BASIL trial findings would have only limited value for us. With only limited time in your day, I recommend focusing primarily (and perhaps solely) on those articles directly applicable to your patient population, and I recommend determining this at the start.

Ask Also, What Are the Outcomes (the O, in the P-I-C-O) Being Studied—Are They Important? Are Any Missing?

It is important to identify whether *all* clinically important outcomes were considered. Many foot/ankle surgical studies still rely heavily on radiographic outcomes due to their inherent convenience. However, it is unlikely that radiographic outcomes, alone, would ever be enough to alter or change the way in which one practices. It is for this very reason, then, that radiographic studies are rarely entertained in our journal club sessions. Similarly, although more and more studies are reporting clinically important outcomes (eg, patient-reported outcome measures [PROMs]), they are not always as careful and complete in depicting the rate(s) of important adverse events and complications.[4] Take note of this. Both are needed to determine the potential benefit (or detriment) of adding a new therapeutic approach.

Finally, Consider How the Treatment Benefits Compare with the Costs and Potential Harms

Before applying and readily adopting a new technology or surgical approach, it is important to weigh the potential costs and harms, as well as any anticipated benefits. This requires an understanding not only of the magnitude of the treatment effect but also of the prevalence of important complications. Readers should have a clear understanding of the major and minor complication rates and not only consider how burdensome the complications are but also consider the additional costs that may be associated with them. To better illustrate this point, I encourage you to consider the results of a recent cost effectiveness analysis our group published looking at the routine use of low-molecular-weight-heparin (LMWH) for venous thromboembolism (VTE) prophylaxis after foot or ankle surgery.[5] Despite assuming a very large therapeutic (actually prophylactic) effect on VTE risk (we assumed a 50% absolute risk reduction with LMWH use), there was no surgery that we examined (ie, ankle fracture ORIF, ankle replacement surgery, hindfoot arthrodesis, or hallux valgus surgery) where routine LMWH use was deemed cost effective from a third party payer's perspective.[5] Without being overly simplistic, this was essentially because the seriousness and costs associated with the infrequent complications with LMWH consistently tipped the scales in favor of no prophylaxis in each of the 4 foot and ankle surgeries we looked at. Although we will not always have the results of a formal cost effectiveness analysis to draw on, we should still critically evaluate the authors' conclusions, considering both the potential harms and costs that are reasonably associated with the therapeutic/intervention in question, and judge it accordingly.

STEP 2: WHAT *ARE* THE RESULTS?
How Large Was the Treatment Effect?

Studies are quick to report statistically significant differences when they exist but it is imperative that the reader (if not the author themselves) put the difference into *clinical perspective*. Some differences are so small that, despite being statistically significant, they would never alter the way in which one practices. However, some differences are quite large and, if precise, would warrant our careful consideration for implementation into clinical and surgical practice. Studies typically report their primary and secondary findings as a rate difference (for dichotomous outcomes) or a mean difference for outcomes measured on a continuous scale. I will provide an example of both.

Assessing the Magnitude of the Treatment Effect When Working with Dichotomous Outcomes

We recently read an article that compared the rate of progression onto ankle Charcot neuroarthropathy after midfoot fusion in 2 groups of patients: those that had concomitant subtalar joint (STJ) arthrodesis at the time of their midfoot fusion and those that did not have concomitant STJ arthrodesis.[6] This is a hot topic, and one of considerable debate. It was published by several authors for whom we have considerable respect. It involved a relatively large cohort of patients, 72 in total, 28 with concomitant STJ fusions and 44 without STJ fusion. With 8 patients in the STJ fusion group going onto ankle Charcot neuroarthropathy by the study's end (event rate: 8/28 = 0.285) and 14 in the no STJ group (event rate 14/44 = 0.318), the authors concluded that the event rates were not the same, Fisher's exact P = .001.[6] They concluded also, that based on this, STJ fusion may be a useful adjunct in midfoot fusion. The problem, of course, is that we are not sure—with only this information—if this technique is truly worthy of our implementation. What we really need to know is, what is the magnitude of the treatment effect and (as was already discussed earlier), what are the costs and potential harms associated with such an approach?

Let us look at our calculations for the magnitude of the treatment effect for the study's primary finding in **Table 1**. As you can see, the treatment (STJ fusion) reduced the risk of progression onto ankle neuroarthropathy by only 10% (RRR = 0.104) relative to that occurring in the control group. Therefore, the magnitude of the treatment effect found in this study is, in fact, not terribly large. To put this another way, using number needed to treat (NNT), you would need to treat 30 people undergoing midfoot reconstruction with a concomitant STJ fusion to prevent one person from progressing onto ankle neuroarthropathy that otherwise would have. If the additional risks and costs associated with added STJ fusion during the index surgery are low, then the modest benefit gained from STJ fusion in halting proximal disease progression may in fact be worth it. If not, the modest benefit likely will not be enough to change practice patterns or recommendations.

Assessing the Magnitude of the Treatment Effect Using Continuous Outcomes

When outcomes are measured on a continuous scale, then the mean difference is typically reported. It is important to closely examine the magnitude of these mean differences to put the treatment effect into perspective, before blindly accepting the authors' conclusions. As a section editor for the *Journal of Foot & Ankle Surgery*, and ad hoc reviewer for other journals, one of the most common pitfalls I see is when authors overstate an observed (ie, statistically significant) mean difference on the visual analog scale (VAS) for pain between their groups, whereas it is still less than 1.0 cm (on a 10-cm scale). These small differences (although possibly statistically significant) do not represent meaningful clinical differences on the VAS pain scale for most conditions. In fact, most studies suggest the minimum clinically important difference (MCID) in VAS pain lies somewhere between 1.0 and 1.5 cm or more.[7] MCIDs have been calculated for many foot/ankle conditions using many of our widely used PROMs at this point, including the various scales within Patient Reported Outcomes Measurement Information System (PROMIS), foot function index, foot and ankle ability measure, foot and ankle outcome scores, and others. If the authors have not taken the time to put the magnitude of their results into perspective, then the reader must attempt to do this before accepting the results at face value.

Next ask, how precise was the estimate of the treatment effect?

Many times, 95% confidence intervals (CIs) will accompany the authors' estimate of the treatment effect. The tighter the interval, the more confidence we have in the stated effect estimate but it is important to remember that in the end, it is still only an estimate. Some studies will even go as far as saying that, "A treatment reduced the risk of an event by [X] times." However, this type of language is probably only reasonable when the CI surrounding the estimate is extraordinarily narrow. Let us look at a recent article our team published looking at the effects of injectable amnion in patients with plantar fasciitis and see how we can put this into practice.[8]

In this study we noticed a 2.3 point mean difference in patient-reported numeric pain rating (NPR) scores for patients with plantar fasciitis treated with an injectable amnion, compared with those treated with only a conventional heel pain treatment protocol during a roughly 3-month observation period (**Table 2**). The effect was in favor of those receiving the amnio injection in the heel. The "2.3" in this instance refers to the *point estimate* for the treatment effect. Although the true improvement in NPR scores seen in the amnio group (compared with the conventionally treated group) is likely close to this value, it is unlikely to be precisely correct. In **Table 2**, you will see that there is a 95% CI accompanying the point estimate. This is the range within which the true treatment effect lies (or would lie) 95% of the time, if we had repeated this study 100 times. Because the 95% CI does not include 0, we can be certain that the mean difference observed is statistically significant when α is set at the 0.05 level. The tighter or narrower the interval, the more certain we are that our reported estimate approximates the truth, and the more appropriate it is then to refer to the point estimate when reporting the magnitude of treatment effect (eg, "we found a 2.3 reduction in NPR scores…"). With CIs that are more wide ranging, however, it is probably more appropriate to simply refer to the fact that there was an observed group difference alone (provided the range for mean difference does not include 0, or the range for a risk estimate does not include 1.0) while placing less emphasis on the actual point estimate obtained. To better illustrate this last point, let us look at how we described the risk of failing nonoperative care by treatment group. As we can see from **Table 2**, 55% of patients receiving conventional heel pain treatment alone underwent plantar fascia surgery, compared with only 7% in the amnio group. This corresponded to an odds ratio of 15.6 (95% CI 3.0 to 27.9).[8] The point estimate (alone) suggests that patients receiving amnio were approximately 15 times more likely to avoid surgery than the comparison group. However, to refer to the magnitude of the amnio effect in this way would be very misleading because the real risk ranges anywhere from 3 (still clinically important) to 28 greater odds as given by the 95% CI. In this study, due to the wide-ranging CIs, we then choose to state only that a difference in rates between the 2 groups was observed while avoiding any reference to the actual magnitude of the risk reduction.

In instances of a *positive study* finding, it is important to look closely at the *lower boundary* of the reported CI. If it is still large enough for the surgeon to recommend the treatment (eg, the −0.82 points we observed on the NPR scale, or being 3.0 times less likely to fail nonoperative treatment), then even despite the uncertainty surrounding the true magnitude of effect, the study results may still be considered more definitive, and it may still be worth adopting the proposed treatment. The same can be said of a *negative study* (one in which the authors conclude that treatment is no better than control therapy). In these instances, look at the *upper limit* of the CI. If the relative risk reduction or mean difference at this upper boundary, if true, is still clinically important, then the study has failed to exclude an important treatment effect.

STEP 3: VALIDITY

Assessment of study validity requires the reader to systematically ask (and answer) 5 additional questions.[2] In answering these questions, you will learn just how well *bias*

Table 2
Measures (in boldface) used to evaluate the precision of the effect estimate

	Amnio (Treatment) Group N = 27	No Amnio (Control) Group N = 27	P Value	Mean Difference (95% CI)	Odds Ratio (95% CI)
NPR score at end of OP – mean (sd)	2.1 (2.3)	4.4 (2.8)	0.004	2.3 (0.82 to 3.7)	–
Failed nonoperative care – count (proportion)	2 (0.07)	15 (0.55)	<0.001	–	15.6 (3.0 to 27.9)

Abbreviations: NPR, numeric pain rating; OP, observation period; sd, standard deviation.

and *confounding* was minimized in the study's conduct and design. These are the 2 primary threats that cloud our interpretation of study findings in lower CLOE studies but, in a well-conducted RCT, these can all but be eliminated. [Note: *"chance,"* commonly referred to as the third threat, is more closely related to sample size and the precision of the magnitude of the treatment effect as described above]. Prospective enrollment of subjects allows for the opportunity to significantly minimize bias and confounding, so do your due diligence and examine how well the authors did.

1. Ask whether the study involved *randomization?* This is such an important part of study design that the CONSORT checklist devotes 3 questions (out of 21 total) just to the quality of the randomization process, including how effective was the random sequence generation, allocation concealment mechanism, and implementation.[9] Most surgical studies in the United States do not involve randomization; so many times the best we can hope for is that the authors took the needed steps to minimize the potential biases and/or confounders that threaten study validity now that randomization is off the table.

2. The next step is determining whether the *groups are equal at the start*. This is determined by examining the distribution of characteristics across the 2 (or more) groups in a table of demographics. You are, at this point, looking to see if any known confounders (eg, stage of disease progression, age, body mass index, activity levels, and so forth) are unequally distributed across the groups at the start. In RCTs, this table will also tell you how well the randomization worked. If the randomization was highly effective (ie, the groups look very similar at the start), you can assume that there is equal distribution *not only* in the known confounders between groups but also, and very importantly, in the equal distribution of the *unknown* confounders. When groups are not equal, then the authors should adjust for these differences in the analysis phase through multivariable modelling. If these differences are not controlled for, then the authors' findings will suffer at least partially from the effects of *residual confounding*. It is common for nonrandomized prospective (and especially retrospective) cohort studies to suffer also from *selection bias*. This occurs when dissimilar groups are selected/enrolled at the start, and subsequently compared.

3. Were the *groups treated equally, aside from the treatment allocation?* Look at the methods section to ensure that the groups had similar follow-up schedules, access to additional treatments, and so forth. When bias creeps in at this level of the study conduct/design, it is referred to as *performance and/or information bias.*

4. Were *all patients who entered the trial/study accounted for?* Moreover, if you are dealing with an RCT, were they analyzed within the groups to which they were randomized? Losses to follow-up should be minimal—preferably less than 20%. One of the primary differentiators of a CLOE 1 and CLOE 2 RCT is having fewer than 20% losses to follow-up. However, if few patients have the outcome of interest, then even small losses to follow-up can bias the results. Patients should be analyzed in the groups to which they were randomized—this is referred to as an "intention-to-treat analysis." When members of the cohort go missing, or are otherwise unaccounted for, this is referred to as *nonresponder or transfer bias*, and is common in foot/ankle studies.

5. Finally, were the *outcome measures and assessments objective and were the patients, clinicians, and assessors kept "blind" to which treatment was being received?* It is ideal if the study is "double-blinded"—that is, both patients and investigators are unaware of treatment allocation. If the outcome is objective (eg, death) then blinding is less critical. If the outcome is subjective (eg, symptoms or

function, like the ACFAS scoring scale[10]) then blinding of the outcome assessor is critical. *Assessment or ascertainment bias* is common among loosely conducted prospective CLOE 3 studies. Other examples of bias at this level include *detection, recall*, and *interviewer bias.*

Although we place a lot of effort into screening and selecting articles for review (Steps 1 and 2), our journal club sessions provide the forum to scrutinize the study's validity openly and objectively (Step 3). This is done in an honest effort to better understand just how reliable the authors' conclusions are. When doing this, it is important to remember that "the final assessment of validity is never a yes-or-no decision. Rather, one can think of validity as a continuum, ranging from strong studies that are very likely to yield an accurate estimate of the treatment effect to weak studies that are very likely to yield a biased estimate."[1] On a good day or session, some of us will start to change the way in which we practice and/or operate almost immediately, and on a bad day, we are left scratching our heads and wondering "who picked this article?!"

DISCLOSURE

The authors have nothing to disclose.

REFERENCES

1. Bhandari M, Guyatt GH, Swiontkowski MF. User's guide to the orthopaedic literature: how to use an article about a surgical therapy. J Bone Joint Surg Am 2001; 83(6):916–26.
2. Centre for Evidence-Based Medicine/University of Oxford. Critical Appraisal Tools. Available at: https://www.cebm.ox.ac.uk/resources/ebm-tools/critical-appraisal-tools. Updated 2023. Accessed June 28, 2023.
3. Adam DJ, Beard JD, Cleveland T, et al. Bypass versus angioplasty in severe ischaemia of the leg (BASIL): multicentre, randomised controlled trial. Lancet 2005;366(9501):1925–34.
4. Fleischer AE, Klein EE, Bowen M, et al. Comparison of combination weil metatarsal osteotomy and direct plantar plate repair versus weil metatarsal osteotomy alone for forefoot metatarsalgia. J Foot Ankle Surg 2020;59(2):303–6.
5. Robinson R, Wirt TC, Barbosa C, et al. Routine use of low-molecular-weight heparin for deep venous thrombosis prophylaxis after foot and ankle surgery: a cost-effectiveness analysis. J Foot Ankle Surg 2018;57(3):543–51.
6. Mateen S, Thomas MA, Jappar A, et al. Progression to hindfoot charcot neuro-arthropathy after midfoot charcot correction in patients with and without subtalar joint arthrodesis. J Foot Ankle Surg 2023;62(4):731–6.
7. Landorf KB, Radford JA, Hudson S. Minimal Important Difference (MID) of two commonly used outcome measures for foot problems. J Foot Ankle Res 2010; 3:7.
8. Matthews M, Betrus CJ, Klein EE, et al. Comparison of regenerative injection therapy and conventional therapy for proximal plantar fasciitis. J Foot Ankle Surg 2023;62(3):469–71.
9. Schulz KF, Altman DG, Moher D. CONSORT 2010 statement: updated guidelines for reporting parallel group randomised trials. BMJ 2010;340:c332.
10. Cook JJ, Cook EA, Rosenblum BI, et al. Validation of the American college of foot and ankle surgeons scoring scales. J Foot Ankle Surg 2011;50(4):420–9.

Narrative Review to Meta-Analysis

A Cookbook Approach to Evidence Synthesis in Surgical Research

Jeremy J. Cook, DPM, MPH, CPH[a,b,*], Tyler Rodericks, DPM[a,b],
Emily A. Cook, DPM, MPH, CPH[a,b]

KEYWORDS

• Evidence synthesis • Meta-analysis • Systematic review • Narrative review

KEY POINTS

- Evidence synthesis is a distilled anthology of the current knowledge related to a particular subject.
- At the upper tiers of study design (systematic review and meta-analysis), evidence synthesis is held in high regard due to methodology transparency and reproducibility.
- Specific methodological choices can influence outcomes, so it is imperative to select many features a priori.

DIFFERENCES IN NARRATIVE REVIEW, SCOPING REVIEW, SYSTEMATIC REVIEW, AND META-ANALYSIS

The preceding articles covered a broad spectrum of clinic trial designs to collect data pertaining to specific patient populations, disease states, and treatments. This article is focused on summarization of the current knowledge base with the expressed goal of guidance toward accurate and complete information about a given topic. Articles which are categorized as evidence synthesis are not actively introducing new data but synthesize the currently available literature into a consensus of topic. Broadly, there are 4 subtypes within this summary domain: (1) narrative review, (2) scoping review, (3) systematic review, and (4) meta-analysis, although technically the meta-analysis is considered a subset of systematic reviews. For the purposes of organization and clarity, they will be treated as distinct research designs in this article. Typically the accepted hierarchy is that meta-analysis is considered the highest tier, followed

a Division of Podiatric Surgery, Department of Surgery, Mount Auburn Hospital, 330 Mount Auburn Street, Suite 519, Cambridge, MA 02138, USA; b Harvard Medical School, Boston, MA, USA
* Corresponding author.
E-mail addresses: jcook2@mah.harvard.edu; jeremycook@post.harvard.edu

Clin Podiatr Med Surg 41 (2024) 291–311
https://doi.org/10.1016/j.cpm.2023.08.002
0891-8422/24/© 2023 Elsevier Inc. All rights reserved.

podiatric.theclinics.com

closely by systematic review, and trailed by the scoping and narrative reviews. This tiering is related to the degree of rigorous framework applied to selecting scientific results and therefore impacts reliability and reproducibility. Regardless of which summary report is implemented, they all fall prey to time. New data are being constantly presented and published, and since these reviews are not updated in real time, they become less accurate over time. According to Shojania 2007, it is estimated that the validity of a summary review is approximately 5.5 years.

Narrative Review

What is a narrative review? If you have ever read an article that summarizes data related to a specific topic, you have seen a narrative review. Many articles in various iterations of the "Clinics series" could be correctly classified as a narrative review. Narrative reviews are significantly vulnerable to selection bias. An easy way to determine if you are looking at a narrative review versus the other aforementioned summary reports is to look for a methods section. If this is missing or anemic, then you can rest assured that you are reading a narrative review. This format relies heavily on the author's opinion of what is relevant to a topic. Authors may opt to omit research which detracts from their objective regardless of quality. For example, an author wishes to demonstrate the expense of intramedullary hammertoe implants and incorporates data from an editorial article for the prices instead of a higher level cohort which cites the specific price of an implant being studied. The discretion of the author drives the inclusion and exclusion of the data available instead of a rigorous a priori structure. Because of this subjective approach, it negatively impacts transparency and reproducibility. These are essential features of high-quality or high-level medical evidence. The reason that randomized controlled trials (RCTs) and meta-analysis are so revered in the research pantheon is because of their inherent reliability. The methods for setting up the experiment are detailed in such a way that outside individuals or teams could evaluate or even repeat the study. In an RCT with the same parameters, the patient sample might be different but the outcomes would likely be very similar if the design is robust and the results are accurately reported. In meta-analysis, this is even more true because a second team could have access to the exact same pool of studies and if the same methods are applied, then the same results should be achieved, hence reproducible. The remaining formats provide escalating structure to reinforce the reliability and reproducibility of research.

Scoping Reviews

The next rung on the evidence synthesis ladder is the scoping review which evolved from the systematic review approach. They can be contrasted to narrative reviews because they include an a priori protocol that applies a structured methodology with transparency to synthesize research. They share several features with systematic reviews but the aims and purposes differ. Scoping reviews aim to provide an overview of the evidence base without a critical appraisal that generates a result related to a specific topic.[1] Munn and colleagues provide an excellent treatise on the salient features of scoping reviews. They propose that if a researcher is "more interested in the identification of certain characteristics/concepts in papers or studies, and in the mapping, reporting or discussion of these characteristics/concepts" than a specific question, then the scoping review format is more appropriate than a systematic review.[1] One of the greatest strengths of scoping reviews is the capacity to systematically identify gaps in the knowledge base to prompt future study. A key difference from the systematic review is that scoping reviews do not include any assessments of bias or methodological limitations of the included evidence. Thus, the quality of the source data is not necessarily equivalent to those studies included in meta-analysis and systematic reviews which often focus on RCTs. The first formalized framework for scoping reviews was described by Arksey and O'Malley in 2005. Since that time, there have been many recommendations regarding iterative changes to methods and reporting. It is this patchwork approach that has diminished the value of scoping reviews within the evidence synthesis domain. Because of the varying and, at times, conflicting standards that constitute the scoping review framework, the reliability is less robust than systematic reviews and meta-analysis. It is our opinion that the Preferred Reporting Items for Systematic reviews and Meta-Analyses (PRISMA)-Extension for Scoping Reviews[2] provides the optimal guidance. Evidence maps are a similar format but are well beyond the scope and purpose of the current article.

Systematic Review

Our next rung on the evidence synthesis ladder is the systematic review. Unlike the narrative review, systematic reviews employ a rigorous framework to summarize a large and complex body of data. As noted earlier, it differs from a scoping review by attempting to answer a focused question that includes evidence with optimization of bias risk. More precisely, the systematic review emphasizes quality over quantity in order to maximize validity. By focusing on a specific question, the systematic review limits incidental linkages in the casual pathway. Further, the systematic review clarifies the strengths and weaknesses of included studies. Regarding treatments, systematic reviews can investigate explicit variations in treatment outcomes as well as highlight generalizability of known intervention effects. Additionally, it is an excellent design for epidemiologic questions such as frequency, risk factors, and prognosis of a disease. Assessment of diagnostic methods/technology is also well-served in the systematic review format.

Meta-Analysis

The final evidence synthesis format to discuss is the meta-analysis study design. This differs from the systematic review by following a similar analytical model but then pool the results from each of the primary studies and reanalyze them to look at the effect of a selected intervention. Unlike a systematic review, where minimization of bias is the central objective, the performance of a meta-analysis requires that the selected primary studies also must be similar enough to justify pooling of the data for additional statistical analysis. Individual studies may be inadequately powered to reject the null hypothesis, whereas the pooled analysis may increase the sensitivity to find smaller differences. This pooled reanalysis is not without potential limitations; results are largely dependent upon quality of the studies as well as the experimental conditions. There must be a certain level of consistency within the studies, or those differences will ultimately nullify the benefits of pooled analysis. The meta-analysis approach conveys a best average estimate of an effect and the uncertainty of that estimate. Formal statistical analysis does not preclude the need for cautious interpretation.

A commonly asked question is "How many studies are needed to perform a meta-analysis?" and the answer is that it depends on the quality of the primary studies and variance in the outcome of those studies. The greater the variance, the more studies are needed to generate an accurate effect estimate. An important consideration is that in a meta-analysis the individual primary study is the unit of analysis and not the patient. That being said, it is generally accepted that a small meta-analysis includes 15 to 20 primary studies. The details of how to perform the relevant steps in a systematic review and meta-analysis will be discussed in the subsequent sections.

A BRIEF PRIMER ON THE CONDUCT OF SYSTEMATIC REVIEWS AND META-ANALYSIS

The first step is to identify a question to be answered by the systematic review. Next, a review of the existent literature must be performed but with strict standards. By definition, all forms of evidence synthesis are retrospective and are vulnerable to those elements of bias. To counter this, a specified a priori protocol must be developed to enable transparency and replicability. The 2 primary protocol elements that must be established a priori are (1) inclusion and exclusion criteria, henceforth referred to as selection criteria and (2) the search strategy. By establishing these constructs in advance, an important source of bias is minimized.

DEVELOPING A RESEARCH QUESTION

A well-focused and well-designed research question is the first and one of the most important components in developing any study and this holds true for systematic reviews and meta-analyses. A frequently encountered pitfall found in many investigations is to lose focus with a slew of questions the researchers attempt to answer in a single study, most of which are not the primary outcome measures by all linguistic or methodologic indications. In reality, many of these additional questions could have constituted their own independent study. That is not to say secondary outcome measures are not valuable or should not be reported, but a high-quality study will maintain focus on the primary outcome for which it was designed and will present secondary outcomes without replacing the primary outcome during the conduct of the study. There are many tools commonly used to help develop or identify a well-designed and narrowly focused research question. One of the most common methods, called the (patient/population, intervention, comparison, outcomes) PICO method, involves answering 4 consecutive questions to help one identify a good question and ultimately a basic framework for a study:[3]

- Patient/population—who is the patient, group, or population being evaluated?
  - That is, (1) men with hallux rigidus or (2) patients with displaced Wb b ankle fractures
- Intervention—what is being done for the patient?
  - That is, (1) First metatarsophalangeal joint fusion or (2) ankle fracture open reduction and internal fixation
- Comparison—what alternative is being considered from the intervention mentioned earlier?
  - That is, (1) First metatarsophalangeal joint hemi-arthroplasty or (2) fracture conservative management with casting
- Outcomes—what specifically are you evaluating between the 2 groups and what do you wish to accomplish or identify?
  - That is, (1) improved pain and function scores or (2) incidence of ankle arthritis with long term follow-up

INCLUSION AND EXCLUSION (SELECTION) CRITERIA

Strategic use of inclusion and exclusion criteria enables researchers to better focus their study and is important for narrowing the range of publications that may be deemed acceptable for inclusion in the review or meta-analysis. Inclusion criteria are specific conditions that must be present within a given study for it to be a part of the analysis, whereas exclusion criteria are specific conditions that, if present, will exclude a given study from being included for analysis.[4,5] For example, if researchers are performing a meta-analysis to assess surgical treatment outcomes in young athletes after acute repair of an Achilles tendon rupture, then they might use "surgical repair <2 weeks after injury" as an inclusion criterion and "patients with neuromuscular disorders" as an exclusion criterion. In this manner, they have excluded studies where the tendon was repaired more than 2 weeks from the date of injury as well as studies evaluating patients who have a neuromuscular condition, both of which may represent a different patient population and act as confounders if included.

Some commonly considered inclusion and exclusion criteria may include the following:

- Dates—to narrow time frames of interest
- Study design—can narrow the types of studies included (ie, RCTs or retrospective studies)
- Exposure—what condition do the participants need to have experienced to be included
- Language—often only studies in the authors' language or languages are included
- Participants—are studies with particular participants desired (ie, children or adults)
- Reported outcomes—is there a particular outcome or outcomes measure that the researchers are interested in
- Types of literature—peer-reviewed or non-peer reviewed literature

Selection criteria must be defensible, meaning that there must be a logical or medically based justification for adoption of the selection criteria. The selection criteria must be applied fairly and equally to all studies that are reviewed. It's important to know that not all evidence is admissible. For instance, experimental studies, regardless of randomization, can and should be included. Non-human studies (animal, bench top, and so forth) should be excluded assuming the objective is for human clinical research. Abstracts presented at conferences are frequently indexed in databases but should not be included because they were never officially published and may not have undergone formal peer review. Similarly, letters to the editor and editorials should be excluded. Research synthesis articles are controversial in terms of acceptability because they increase the risk of double counting studies. One of the predominant rules of admissible evidence is that no new data can be introduced by the investigators, meaning that proprietary or unpublished data cannot be included for any reason. Observational and epidemiologic studies may be acceptable depending on the study question. Case series are typically excluded but may be acceptable in rare cases.

PERFORMING A LITERATURE SEARCH

The Internet and widespread collaboration have enabled comprehensive searches to a degree never before experienced by researchers. Bibliographic searches that previously took years now take moments. Detailed below is a sampling of databases that effectively span the breadth and width of medical knowledge with some limitations. For instance, MEDLINE is an excellent database; however, it cannnot access articles published before 1965. Such limitations require caution to ensure appropriate studies are not excluded and require that the investigators understand the limits of where they search. Beyond these online repositories also consider some additional search methods. Cross-checking citations or "snowballing" is where the investigator does a title review of articles listed in the bibliography of a pertinent study to identify additional potential studies. Another option is to speak to other investigators in the field to ascertain if they are familiar with other studies that might not be indexed in the typical databases. Exclusion from many databases occurs when there is no English translation available, but they may still contain relevant data. It is noteworthy that excluding non-English publications is considered acceptable. Two distinct analyses of RCTs used in systematic reviews and meta-analysis concluded that use of English-language as an inclusion criterion resulted in no evidence of systematic bias.[6,7] It's important to understand that the inclusion of high-quality non-English trials did improve the precision of the pooled estimates and therefore still have value. Yet another issue is that some investigators may generate multiple publications from a single study. In these instances, it's considered appropriate to utilize the most recent publication, the largest publication, or the highest quality publication when this issue arises. This minimizes double counting and the distortion of data. A sample of commonly used databases is listed below.

PubMed

This is a search engine that primarily accesses the MEDLINE database as well as some additional resources maintained by the US National Library of Medicine. It is free to use and does provide access to some free full-text articles. The database mostly includes English articles.

Embase

Stands for Excerpta Medica Database. This is a subscription database that includes everything in the MEDLINE database as well as roughly an additional 7 million biomedical and pharmacologic records.

Web of Science

This is a subscription-based service that uses scientific citation indexing to search multiple databases.[8]

Ovid

This is a search engine that hosts multiple databases. Essentially it provides advanced search features that can be used/applied to search multiple databases to which a subscription is held. This allows the use of a consistent set of advanced search features to search multiple databases simultaneously. An Ovid subscription must be held for each database being searched.[9]

Additional resources include Google Scholar, Scopus, EBSCO, ClinicalTrials.gov, the Cochrane Library, and Cochrane Central Register of Controlled Trials.

DEVELOPING SEARCH TERMS

A database search using keywords is likely the most common method used by the majority of individuals accessing a database to search a given topic. Utilizing keywords or a free text search will identify research containing the search terms in the titles, abstracts, or other fields that are available in the database. However, this may not represent the most effective strategy to identify all literature on a given topic. Databases are indexed utilizing "controlled vocabulary," which is functionally a hierarchical family tree using progressively narrower standardized terms into which articles are categorized.[10] Identifying the controlled vocabulary used in a database and implementing the controlled vocabulary into a search enable a search to return the entire category of literature that is indexed under the controlled vocabulary term that is used. Database search engines allow controlled vocabulary search terms to be "exploded" which means all indexed literature that falls within subcategories of the searched term will also be included in the search. In most instances the broadest relevant controlled vocabulary term should be used and exploded terms should be included to ensure all literature within the category is being captured. A well-designed literature search will strategically combine these 2 methods, narrowing a search to a standardized subcategory with controlled vocabulary and then searching for free text terms or keywords within that category.[11]

A range of terms should be used when adding free text to a search to be as comprehensive as possible. Synonyms, acronyms, various forms of a word, and spelling variants should all be considered for potential search terms.[11] Some search engines allow various strategies to broaden a searched term to include more of these variants. For example, truncation can often be used to capture multiple forms of the same word, and wildcards can often be used to capture spelling variants on a given word. Proximity operators can often be used to identify literature that contains the search terms up to a given number of words from each other within the paper (**Table 1**).

ELIMINATING DUPLICATES

Identification and elimination of duplicate literature is important, particularly for meta-analysis where duplicate studies have significant potential to introduce biases into the results. Some search engines (ie, Ovid) and citation managing software (ie, Mendeley) have deduplication functions to aid in this process; however, these functions may not be perfect to have the potential to remove false duplicates, which may be detrimental to the study as it may lead to exclusion of relevant studies.[12] There are also some duplicates that such a function may miss, as a duplicate is not just represented by an identical publication but can also be separate publications reporting on different outcomes or time points for the same original study.

There are multiple strategies to aid in manually identifying and eliminating potential duplicates. These include comparing trial identification numbers or other unique study identifiers, comparison of author names, comparison of the location the trial took place, specific details of the methodology, intervention, number of participants, baseline data, or date and duration of the study. For those publications that represent multiple reports about the same study, the data should be collated and the primary report to be used for study results must be selected.[11]

DATA EXTRACTION OVERVIEW

An often-overlooked part of the search methodology is the reporting of said search methods. It's important to include a list of the excluded studies and why. Include operational definitions for both explanatory and response variables. Each selected study should be assessed independently by at least 2 evaluators to ensure precise data

Table 1			
Examples of free text search methods			
	Truncation	**Wildcards**	**Proximity Operators**
Search	Run*	Woman	gait adj1 device
Return	Runs, Running, runner, runt, run	Woman, Women	Gait-training device, gait-stabilizing device, device-assisting gait

* Is the character that signifies that all possbile matches are requested.

extraction. The final report should include a measure of inter-extractor reliability such as a kappa score. Data extraction can be a time consuming process and should be explicitly addressed in an organized fashion that is unbiased and reproducible. Gøtzsche and colleagues reported that in 63% of 27 meta-analyses they studied, at least 1 study had an extraction error that invalidated the meta-analysis.[13] There are 2 key components to effective and organized data extraction.

Data Collection Forms

The first is for the reviewers to develop data collection forms. Data collection forms are a tool that enables data extractors to obtain necessary information or data from the studies being assessed in a structured and organized fashion. These forms are typically comprised of a set of questions addressing each specific data point that is to be collected and are best designed with fixed selectable responses known as coded responses (except where numerical data is to be inputted). Sample data points that might be found on such a form may include study design, level of evidence, demographic data, number of participants, results, outcome scoring systems, outcome scores, length of follow-up, and so on. All data fields should be filled for each study from which data will be extracted, and the coded responses should also include options such as "unreported," "other, specify," or "unclear" to account for studies for which the data does not fit the other selectable coded responses. Each form should also include space for who extracted the data.[11]

Separate collection forms may also be considered for various components of the data collection process, such as first using one form to identify studies to include or exclude and then using a second from for data extraction from an individual study that was included. A well-designed data collection form will collect sufficient data to preclude the need to return to the original studies after the data extraction process is complete. Data collection forms should undergo pilot testing to ensure they collect all necessary data in the appropriate format to allow for later analysis. This way necessary revisions can be made prior to final distribution and initiation of the data extraction process. For smaller studies, distribution of paper or electronic data collection forms may be sufficient for organization of the extracted data; however, for large scale studies data management systems may be required for effective collation and organization of the extracted data.[11]

Data Extraction

After data collection forms have been developed, pilot tested, and finalized, they can be distributed to the reviewers who will be performing data extraction. It is advisable that extraction be performed independently by multiple reviewers to reduce extraction errors as well as the introduction of potential biases from reviewers. A protocol for handling discrepancies in the extracted data should be in place, and extraction forms from multiple reviewers should then be combined into a single form for each study. Multiple publications for multiple reports of the same study should also be collated into a single form for that study. Data extraction is largely a manual process requiring reviewers to read the studies of interest to identify the data to be extracted. The use of Portable Document Format search functions or automated systems may be able to aid to data extraction; however, these methods still have the potential to miss data points, and the completeness and accuracy of data extracted by these methods must be verified.[11]

Software-based data extraction tools such as WebPlotDigitizer[14] may be particularly helpful for numeric data that is only presented in graphical charts or figures, as this data is not as accurately obtained by visual estimation. Additional calculations may also be necessary for some numerical data that is extracted from a study in order to fill each numerical data field on the data collection form.

Publication Bias

A trend that astute researchers will notice is that the vast majority of articles that get published report outcomes which statistically affirm the hypothesis of a clinical trial as opposed to the smaller fraction of publications reporting negative outcomes or lack of support for the hypothesis. Hedin and colleagues defined it more concisely as the "tendency to publish only results that are statistically or clinically significant."[15] This is referred to as publication bias because many investigators may not wish to pursue the time-consuming process of peer review and the study results go unpublished. This bias is also called the "file drawer problem" because the data languish in a computer or desk never to see the light of day. This is important because exclusion of this missing negative data exaggerates the estimates of intervention. In other words, it makes the reported proportion, relative risk (RR), or odds ratio inaccurate by inflating the results away from reality. In our opinion, the best method for minimizing publication bias is to search registries, contact other investigators in the field of interest, perform funnel plots of your data, and finally make adjustments with your statistical analyses. As noted earlier, searching study registries such as ClinicalTrials.gov can identify studies in progress and pilot studies to see if negative data failed to proceed to publication. Contacting investigators listed on registered but unpublished studies may help identify those gaps in knowledge. Our preferred method for assessing the presence of publication bias is the performance of a funnel plot when selection criteria generate more than 10 studies to be analyzed. The reliability of this technique is challenged when there are 10 or fewer studies in a meta-analysis.[16] It is generally accepted that if the funnel plot is asymmetrical then the likelihood of missing data is high; however, there are other sources of asymmetry that are legitimate. Contour-enhanced meta-analysis funnel plots as reported by Peters and colleagues offer a more in-depth technique for differentiating the probability of these alternative causes of asymmetry.[17]

Quality of Included Studies

The axiom "garbage in, garbage out" holds true to any research project, but meta-analyses are particularly sensitive to this issue. The inclusion of low-quality studies can diminish or exaggerate the calculated effect estimate of the topic. For example, if a low-quality study includes 200 patients while the remaining trials are high-quality but only include 50 patients each, the impact of the large, flawed study distorts the validity of the effect estimate. That is just one example; in reality, several small studies could similarly invalidate the study. That is why establishing a method for assigning quality scores to your included studies a priori is critical for assessment later in your analysis. We usually include a section for quality score or variables we designate as related to quality on our data collection forms. Quality-related variables can be used to help explain heterogeneity as well as enable investigators to conduct sensitivity analysis later on. Features commonly used in experimental studies for judging quality include study design (RCTs vs cohorts vs case-control), randomization success, intention-to-treat versus per-protocol analysis, presence of blinding, length of follow-up, and loss to follow-up. Observational and epidemiologic studies have some overlap but also include differences in exposure and how the outcomes were measured. In our meta-analysis of first metatarsophalangeal implants, we designated studies that were prospective, larger, and had low proportions of lost to follow-up as higher quality to perform sensitivity analysis. At the discretion of the investigators, implementation of formal quality instruments can be used. One such example is the Jadad Quality Score for RCT, which assigns a point value to features of the study in question.[18] If the total points exceed the designated threshold, then the study is considered high-quality. Another more comprehensive assessment tool is the CONSORT (Consolidated Standards of Reporting Trials) protocol which uses a 25-item checklist and a flow diagram to assess RCT quality.[19] It's a free resource available at www.consort-statement.org. A major limitation of such scales is that they are a generic view of quality and can overemphasize study structure instead of variables that are truly impactful to the topic being investigated.

The risk of bias (RoB) table consolidates the assessment of bias of primary studies selected for the systematic review.[20] The RoB 2 tool offered by Cochrane is a commonly administered option for summarizing these findings. Potential sources of bias are highlighted and presented using a colored circle containing a "+," "-," and a "?" representing a low RoB, a high RoB, and an inconclusive RoB, respectively. The sources of bias included in these tables are at the discretion of the investigators with regard to those most relevant to the review. A sample assessment can be seen in **Fig. 1**. The tool can be accessed at https://sites.google.com/site/riskofbiastool/welcome/rob-2-0-tool/current-version-of-rob-2.

Flowchart of data extraction
With the steps detailed in the previous sections completed, the investigators have fully extrapolated all relevant data. As noted before, the foundations of systematic review and meta-analysis are transparency and reproducibility. Simply stating that the remaining studies meet selection criteria is adequate but not optimal. Instead collaborative researchers that reported the CONSORT protocol included a flow diagram detailing the progressive phases of the trial being assessed. This has been heavily adapted to systematic reviews and meta-analyses by noting decision points where studies were selected for inclusion. It starts with the number of articles generated by the primary search in the various databases, then it presents the number of citations retrieved, the number of articles subjected to a title screening, abstract review, and full article review ultimately resulting in the total number of articles meeting selection criteria. Throughout the diagram, the number of articles removed due to duplications and the a priori exclusion criteria are also detailed. A sample chart can be seen in **Fig. 2**.[21] An online resource for this is available at https://www.eshackathon.org/software/PRISMA2020.html.

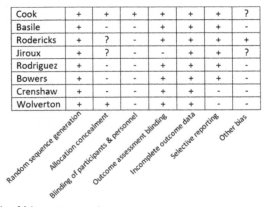

Cook	+	+	+	+	+	+	?
Basile	+	-	-	+	+	+	-
Rodericks	+	?	-	+	+	+	+
Jiroux	+	?	-	-	+	+	?
Rodriguez	+	-	-	+	+	+	-
Bowers	+	-	-	+	+	+	-
Crenshaw	+	-	-	+	+	-	-
Wolverton	+	+	-	+	+	-	-

Random sequence generation / Allocation concealment / Blinding of participants & personnel / Outcome assessment blinding / Incomplete outcome data / Selective reporting / Other bias

Fig. 1. Example risk of bias assessment.

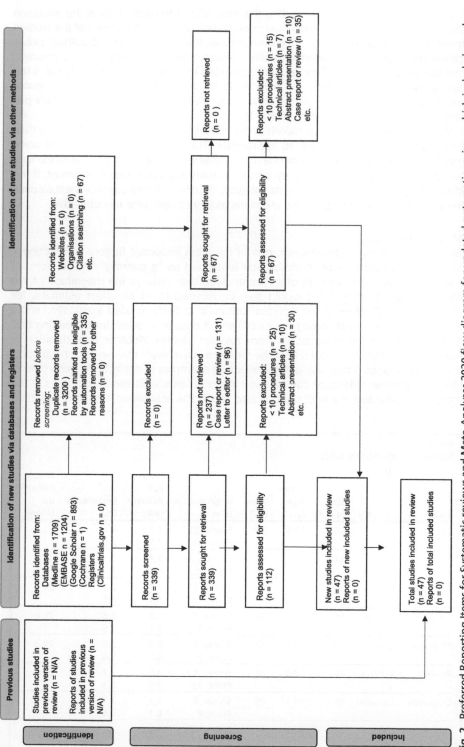

Fig. 2. Preferred Reporting Items for Systematic reviews and Meta-Analyses 2020 flow diagram for updated systematic reviews which included searches of databases, registers, and other sources. (*Adapted From:* Page MJ, McKenzie JE, Bossuyt PM, Boutron I, Hoffmann TC, Mulrow CD, et al. The PRISMA 2020 statement: an updated guideline for reporting systematic reviews. BMJ 2021;372:n71. doi: 10.1136/bmj.n71.)

An effective method for presenting the data related to each study is the evidence table. This is a highly organized visual presentation of pertinent features of the studies meeting the selection criteria. It's common to list the study name (lead author), publication date, study population and size, design, intervention/exposure, outcomes, metatamer, and so forth. This is usually included in the body of the article but if the size is too excessive, it may be included in the appendices. From an investigator perspective, it aids with organizing data in a logical way and can help to identify potential sources of heterogeneity (**Table 2**).

With the preceding steps completed, the investigator may begin summarizing their findings and draw conclusions as appropriate. The discussion should include commentary on the quality of the evidence and an assessment of the limitations of the systematic review, particularly as they pertain to methodological bias abatement. If the study design was intended as a meta-analysis, then the following sections will discuss the differences and the additional steps necessary to complete this objective.

Meta-analysis focus

When performing a meta-analysis, one of the most important factors is selecting a clearly defined metamer. A metameter is defined as "a quantity derived from an observation, and independent of all parameters, that conveys the magnitude of the phenomenon observed."[22] It would also be referred to as an effect estimate, for example, the RR of recurrent Achilles rupture in patients treated surgically versus conservatively. When choosing the metameter it should be consistent, meaning that it is present and easily extracted from relevant studies. Another consideration is ease of interpretation; does it reflect the outcome in a relevant manner? For binary outcomes, RRs, odds ratios, risk difference are all examples of acceptable metameters. Means and mean difference can be used as continuous variables. Regardless of the metameter selected, it's important to also report the associated standard deviation

Table 2
Sample of an evidence table

Study	Country	Size (n = *)	Mean Age (yr)	Male (%)	Intervention (n = *)	Return Full Activity (wk)	Recurrence (%)	Mean Follow-up (Mon)
Cook	USA	62	50.5	20	Screw: 31	7.2	2.1	61.4
					Plate: 31	7.1	2.9	
Basile	USA	44	49.6	18	Screw: 22	5.3	3	48.2
					Plate: 22	6.1	1	
Rodericks	Germany	20	48.7	17	Screw: 10	7.5	2.2	24.3
					Plate: 10	7.9	4.7	
Jiroux	France	14	52	39	Screw: 7	7.1	2.8	26.8
					Plate: 7	7.1	3.6	
Rodriguez	USA	18	54.7	22	Screw: 9	6.3	3.9	29.3
					Plate: 9	6.9	5.6	
Bowers	Austria	26	50.3	18	Screw: 13	7.5	3.2	30.2
					Plate: 13	7.9	4.3	
Crenshaw	Canada	16	55.1	25	Screw: 8	7.7	2.4	44.6
					Plate: 8	8.1	2.6	
Wolverton	UK	24	52.9	21	Screw: 12	6.2	1.3	36.1
					Plate: 12	5.9	2.5	

because this reflects the precision that each study provides regarding that variable. This is relevant since greater variance in an estimate leads to wide confidence intervals which mean less precision. This can help with deciding how much weight a given study deserves mathematically. The concept of combing data is a complex one and due to the constraints of this article must be overly-simplified. Vote counting and combination of P-values are 2 infrequently used methods due to their lack of sophistication. On the opposite end of the spectrum is the Bayesian model which is so mathematically sophisticated that interpretation becomes difficult. More commonly a pooled analysis whereby all studies meeting selection criteria generate an average metatamer that is treated as the numerator and then divided by the number of studies in the denominator, then all studies are given equal weight. This is simple and unbiased but very inefficient. This is because each study likely has different sample sizes and variable precision. To adjust for this, you can instead use fixed effects weights which provide a calculated weighted average of the metatamer and the variance. The benefit here is that the result is weighting proportional to the precision of the study. The downside is that it makes the assumption that the included studies are very similar and the only real source of variation is size and the randomization of the sampling (eg, different population or site). For example, you have 5 studies looking at incidence of recurrence as reflected by average hallux valgus angle after surgery. The bell curve generated for each of these studies looks very similar and the mean recurrence of each study falls on this distribution. Because fixed effect models assume a relatively uniform distribution of the same effect (hallux valgus angle as recurrence), it makes observing a statistically significant difference (P-value equal to 0.05 or lower) easier to achieve. That sounds great but may be potentially very inaccurate. Consider the same study but recurrence is now defined by hallux valgus angle in 2 studies, sesamoid position in 1 study, and intermetatarsal angle in 2 studies. They are assessing parameters of recurrence but in ways that the bell curves look very different from one another. In this instance a random effects model is more appropriate. In this approach, the calculations treat the studies as if they provide an estimate that has slightly different parameters, population, and design. As a result, the model assumes a normal distribution of the true parameter "recurrence" as generated by those 5 studies estimating recurrence in slightly different ways. The effect size for each study is assumed to be from a normal distribution of effect across the studies. The random effects model is considered more conservative because it assumes variability across studies yielding a wider confidence interval which makes observing a statistically significant difference (P-value equal to 0.05 or lower) more difficult to achieve. Without getting into the math directly, the choice between fixed and random effects modeling can be summarized as follows: if there is no single "true" parameter but instead the "truth" is dependent on the details of the selected studies, then a random effects model is the best solution. If the investigator can justify a single "true" parameter and that the studies are effectively clones but with a different population then a fixed effects model can be reported. In reality, a fixed effects model is very difficult to justify. Most programs that perform meta-analysis generate fixed and random effects models simultaneously; if they provide different qualitative answers, then you have a significant problem that requires re-verification of the extrapolated data.

Forest plots

Forest plots are a visual summary of each primary study's contribution. Although the output may vary based upon the program used to generate it, there are some constants that should be discussed for interpretation guidance. In this example (**Fig. 3**),

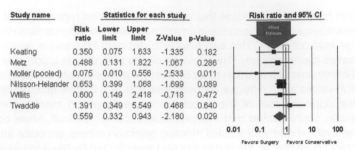

Study name	Statistics for each study					Risk ratio and 95% CI
	Risk ratio	Lower limit	Upper limit	Z-Value	p-Value	
Keating	0.350	0.075	1.633	-1.335	0.182	
Metz	0.488	0.131	1.822	-1.067	0.286	
Moller (pooled)	0.075	0.010	0.556	-2.533	0.011	
Nilsson-Helander	0.653	0.399	1.068	-1.699	0.089	
Willits	0.600	0.149	2.418	-0.718	0.472	
Twaddle	1.391	0.349	5.549	0.468	0.640	
	0.559	0.332	0.943	-2.180	0.029	

Fig. 3. Sample of forest plot.

RR of re-rupture is compared in studies with surgical versus conservative management of Achilles tendon rupture. The first column typically includes the lead author (or study designation) and year published. Each study is given a row that represents the effect estimate, sample size, and a line running through it that represents the confidence interval around the estimate. The size of the square can be uniform or proportional to the sample size. The Nilsson-Helander study has many more patients than the Twaddle study. Nilsson-Helander also has narrower confidence intervals while Moller has very wide confidence intervals, and therefore more variance. The red diamond represents the combined results calculated during the meta-analysis process. The orange box encompasses the line of no effect. In this instance, the line of no effect starts at "1" but it can also begin at "0" depending on the study design. If the diamond makes contact with or overlaps the line of no effect, there is not an observed statistically significant difference between groups. Although the diamond appears to be in contact with the line of no effect, we can confirm this is a scale issue since the combined results upper confidence interval is 0.943. In this instance, the combined results show that surgery has a reduced risk of re-rupture.

HETEROGENEITY

An assessment of heterogeneity across the range of studies included in a meta-analysis is critical for interpreting the potential significance of meta-analysis findings. Ideally, all included studies would measure the same effect as one another. In other words, they would be designed such that all confounding variables are equivalently controlled so the input and output data would be directly representative of the same measure between the comparative relationships being evaluated in each respective study. In this theoretic ideal circumstance, all variation in the findings between studies would be due to random chance since all other potentially contributing factors are equivalently controlled. In reality, not all studies are identical. There can be clinical, methodological, or statistical differences between studies and each of these differences introduces the possibility that different studies evaluating the same comparative relationships are not actually measuring the same thing. They are instead only measuring nuanced variations of an apparently similar relationship.[11]

For example, suppose there are 2 RCTs being used in a meta-analysis to evaluate surgical site infection rates when using one antibiotic for surgical prophylaxis versus another antibiotic. One study may be composed of a primarily diabetic population whereas the other has no diabetics (clinical difference), one study may follow a different protocol for randomization than the other (methodological difference), and one study may statistically handle dropouts differently than the other (statistical difference). On the surface these studies appear to have the same theoretic aim and are reporting on the same comparative outcomes; however, the populations, methods, and statistics being used all differ and may be causative of nonrandom differences in the final results or measured effect that each study identified. In essence, these nonrandom differences occur because the studies in question are not actually making identical comparisons. As a result, it is also less reliable to then compare the findings of these 2 studies to one another in a meta-analysis. One might say it's a comparison of apples and oranges due to the heterogeneity between the 2 studies.

As can be presumed, this potentially presents a substantial problem for researchers doing a meta-analysis because no 2 studies will ever be evaluating truly identical effects. A small degree of heterogeneity is expected and even considered acceptable in a meta-analysis as a result; however, the presence and extent of heterogeneity affects the extent to which generalizable conclusions can be developed. If too much heterogeneity exists, the data from the systematic review may not be suitable for meta-analysis. Multiple statistical models exist to assess the fraction of effects size variation that can be attributed to heterogeneity. A few common ones are described in the following paragraphs.

- Chi^2 test: Assesses if the difference in results is attributable to random chance alone. A high chi-squared value suggests heterogeneity or a non-random cause of the observed difference. The P-value that is frequently reported is the probability that the calculated chi-squared value was by random chance based on a given degrees of freedom (number of studies minus 1). The presence of heterogeneity is, therefore, defined by whether the P-value value falls below a probability threshold deemed significant by the researchers (ie, $P < .10$). The result is a binary indication of the presence or absence of heterogeneity. One of the disadvantages is that the test has low power to detect heterogeneity in a meta-analysis with few studies or studies with small sample sizes. As a result, a high or low chi-squared value may not accurately reflect the presence of heterogeneity. The converse is also true, as the test has high power to detect a potentially inconsequential degree of heterogeneity if there are many studies included in the meta-analysis. The test does not provide an assessment of the extent to which heterogeneity is present.[11]

- Q test: First defined by Cochrane in 1954, this has historically been one of the most common ways to assess heterogeneity in a meta-analysis.[23] The test assumes a null hypothesis that the included studies are all measuring the same thing. Under this assumption, the calculated Q value is theoretically expected to be equal to the degrees of freedom (number of studies minus 1); however, some variability is allowed due to random variation. If the Q value is a lot larger than expected, then the null hypothesis is rejected and heterogeneity is considered to be present. In other words, it's likely the included studies are not measuring quite the same thing.[24] If the null hypothesis is not rejected, the study typically utilizes a fixed effect statistics model which assumes variability in the data is only due to sampling error. If the null hypothesis is rejected, the study will typically utilize a random effects statistics model, which will account better for intra-study and inter-study variability. It suffers from the same disadvantages as the chi-squared test as it has low power to detect heterogeneity if there are only a few studies included and high power to detect inconsequential heterogeneity with many studies included. This may lead the researchers to make an incorrect selection of the most appropriate statistics model to be used.[23] The Q test also does not inform the extent to which heterogeneity is present. For example, a meta-analysis of 6 primary studies generate heterogeneity assessment with a Q of 15.9 ($P = .007$) would show substantial heterogeneity but the interpretation is more difficult.

- I^2 test: The I-squared test is a calculation elaborating upon the calculated Q value in an attempt to subsequently quantify the extent to which heterogeneity exists between studies. The resultant I-squared value represents a percentage of the variability in the effect sizes that can be attributed to heterogeneity rather than chance. Essentially, a value of 0 would mean all variability in the effects size is due to sampling error whereas a value of 40%, for example, would mean 40% of the variability is due to heterogeneity. It is commonly interpreted that a value of 0% to 40% may not be important, 30% to 60% represents moderate heterogeneity, 50% to 90% represents substantial heterogeneity, and 75% to 100% represents considerable heterogeneity. The importance of the I-square value is still dependent on whether the magnitude and direction of effects are not inconsequential as well as the strength of evidence for heterogeneity such as that which is suggested by a P-value or I^2 confidence interval.[11] Disadvantages include considerable uncertainty in the I-squared value when a low number of studies are included.[25]

Now that the presence of heterogeneity has been quantified, there are a variety of methods for dealing with it in the context of analysis, and prudence dictates that since heterogeneity is a common occurrence, the investigators should attempt to define these sources a priori and specify plans for abatement. As noted earlier, use of the random effects model for combining data inherently assumes the presence of heterogeneity and usefully produces the Q test statistical and I^2 test. A popular and relatively easy method for addressing heterogeneity is via subgroup and sensitivity analysis. Subgroups can be assigned based upon logical sources of heterogeneity and include populations, interventions, exposures, dosing, study quality, study design, between or within study groups as well as many other variables that may logically contribute to variance between primary studies. Analysis of variance and F tests effectively make comparisons between subgroups. For continuous variables, a meta-regression can produce effect estimates as they relate to other qualities of the patients.

INTERPRETATION OF RESULTS

Correct interpretation of a study's results depends heavily on an understanding of the statistical analyses that were performed and an understanding of limitations that may impact the study. A confidence interval is a range around a measured effect in which we can estimate the true effect actually lies with a given percentage of confidence. The chi^2 test is reported as a P-value that is compared against an arbitrary probability threshold for significance (meaning the effect did not occur by random chance) and functions hand in hand with the confidence interval. For example, if the threshold is set at 0.05, then the confidence interval will be 95%. Essentially this means a P-value less than 0.05 for a given estimated effect would indicate with 95% certainty that the range of values that may represent the true effect are all above the chosen probability threshold. It is important to understand that significance via a low P-value does not indicate that a treatment has an important benefit. It only indicates that the treatment effect lies beyond the chosen threshold for which the effect can be attributable to random chance. Magnitude of effect must also be assessed to identify benefit. A point estimate (ie, odds ratios, hazard ratios) is an estimate of the magnitude and direction of data. Taken in conjunction with its confidence interval, this can be useful to assess whether the treatment effect had sufficient magnitude to be considered important. For example, if a 10-point American Orthopaedic Foot and Ankle Society score improvement is needed for a particular treatment to be considered beneficial and a meta-analysis had an estimate of a 20-point improvement with a confidence interval of 95% that the true improvement was between 15 to 25 points, then it could be concluded that the treatment was beneficial since the range of possible true values all exceed the 10-point threshold. If the confidence interval for the same 20-point estimate indicated a possible true value range of 5 to 35 points, then one may conclude the treatment is probably beneficial but they cannot do so with as much certainty because there is a probability that the true value lies below the 10-point threshold needed for the treatment to be beneficial.[11]

Additional methods that are sometimes used to express results of a meta-analysis may include number needed to treat or RR reduction. The number needed to treat is a calculated estimation of how many patients need to receive a given intervention in order for 1 additional patient to experience a given effect from it relative to the patients in the comparative group. RR reduction represents a percentage reduction relative to overall risk. For example, if there is a 2% risk of an event occurring and treatment reduces that risk to 1%, then the RR reduction is 50%.[11]

DRAWING CONCLUSIONS

With the additional steps of qualitative analysis, overall summary, and heterogeneity identification and management completed, the investigator may summarize their findings and draw conclusions. As noted throughout this article, consideration of selected primary study quality is imperative. It's important to remember to comment on the quality of evidence and how it relates to the strength of the recommendation. Although treatment "X" might be the numerically superior treatment, other factors such as cost, availability, and side effects might diminish its strength of recommendation. A discussion of publication bias can contextualize the likelihood of exaggeration of the effect estimate. Yet another consideration is the robustness of the estimate, as discussed earlier the choice of statistical model does impact the validity of the analysis. Sensitivity analyses that use sub-analysis of designated high-quality studies will directly challenge robustness, as does the one-study–removed method which can determine if a single study is driving the results. Next, generalizability should be commented on, specifically as it relates to the meta-analysis results applying to the population of interest. This requires evaluation of the demographics and characteristics of patients in the primary studies and determining if they are an adequate representation of the population of interest. This matters because it determines if the meta-analysis results can be extrapolated in a universal or limited manner to that population. When presenting information related to epidemiologic studies, there is the added requirement that the primary studies propose a causal relationship. Finally, the presence of any unexplained heterogeneity should be presented as well as the author's attempt to minimize its impact.

EFFECTIVE EXTRAPOLATION

The results of a meta-analysis or systematic review have the greatest potential for benefit when a reader or researcher can extrapolate the findings to their clinical practice or future research. Effective extrapolation often involves drawing upon the entire body of literature, knowledge, and experience relevant to the study's subject in order to generate an integrated understanding of the study's potential implications upon that practice as a whole. Extrapolation to clinical practice often begins with identifying potential ways the study may change one's practice based solely on the aims and research questions being asked in the study.

Next, the effectiveness and reliability with which the study addressed the aims and research questions that were posed can be assessed. Answering a few questions can be helpful in this assessment: Is the methodology appropriate and are there any inherent methodologic limitations that may impact the reliability of the results? Are there evident biases that may impact the results? To what extent is heterogeneity potentially prohibitive to drawing strong generalized conclusions? Do the results provide the necessary information to answer the research questions? And finally after determining the results to have sufficient reliability, they can be considered for implementation in the context of one's own practice and experience. This often involves weighing risks and benefits of the intervention in question, goals of care for the affected patients, evaluation of whether the study is generalizable to the patient population one treats, technical factors that may impact implementation, and many other aspects of care that may go beyond the scope of what was specifically addressed by the meta-analysis.

Extrapolation to future research often involves the identification of remaining questions that were not answered in the present analysis, or weak points within the available body of literature that could be addressed by well-designed studies in the future. Many research questions also arise from the potential implications for clinical practice that were previously identified.

REPORTING GUIDELINES AND ASSESSMENT TOOLS

The complexity of this topic is evident in the preceding article and the opportunities to commit an error are numerous. Early reported meta-analyses were often found to be incomplete or flawed. In an effort to minimize this occurrence, an international collaboration of researchers developed guidance for reporting meta-analysis of RCTs with the Quality of Reporting of Meta-analysis (QUORUM) consensus statement. In 2005, these guidelines were updated to include the systematic review format as well. This new iteration of QUORUM was designated PRISMA and this was updated once again in 2020.[21,26] The PRISMA statement provides a highly detailed checklist and the flow diagram that can be accessed for free at prisma-statement.org. PRISMA guidelines are intended to increase the reliability of results reported by systematic reviews and meta-analysis which include RCTs.

Given that the early QUORUM working group concluded that the reporting of RCTs was flawed and required guidance, it only made sense that non-RCTs were given guidance as well. Observational study designs (case-control, cohort, cross-section, and so forth) are the most common designs in clinical research and almost two-thirds of systematic reviews include these study designs. It has been reported that upwards of 90% of surgical research is based on observational studies.[27] As noted in prior articles, observational study designs are far more vulnerable to bias but also are more likely to be a source of heterogeneity due to the relatively low structural rigor that is more typically associated with RCTs. Given that podiatric surgery is just as restricted in the performance of RCTs as any other surgical specialty, it's essential to understand that our published systematic reviews will rely heavily on observational data. In 2000, the Centers for Disease Control and Prevention funded a group of experts to publish the Meta-analysis of Observational Studies in Epidemiology (MOOSE) consensus statement.[28] This guidance was similarly updated in 2021.[27] The objective of MOOSE guidelines is to safeguard meta-analyses using observational studies from sources of bias, optimizing quality of primary studies, and improve reporting of results. The exhaustive checklist covers 6 distinct reportable domains: background (6), search strategy (10), methods (4), criteria (4), results (3), discussion (3), and conclusions (4).

Detailing each of these 34-points is beyond the objective of this article but many of the relevant elements are discussed throughout its content; however, the checklist can be accessed for free at elsevier.com/__data/promis_misc/ISSM_MOOSE_Checklist.pdf. Despite its comprehensive nature, this guidance will not completely demonstrate how to conduct a meta-analysis using observational studies nor does it include a study protocol for data extraction. MOOSE is most effective when it is being used to evaluate a meta-analysis or systematic review, and this can be done by the investigators prior to publications, peer reviewers, editors, and the general readership.

The original PRISMA and MOOSE guidelines were more concerned with the primary studies as a source of bias. As these forms of evidence synthesis have become more widespread, research has demonstrated many sources of bias in systematic reviews and more appraisal tools have been introduced. A MeaSurement Tool to Assess systematic Reviews (AMSTAR-2)) is another such tool that can be accessed at http://www.amstar.ca/docs/AMSTAR%202-Guidance-document.pdf.[29] It is primarily focused on overall quality and flawed conduct of the data synthesis for health care interventions. Yet another assessment tool is the Risk Of Bias In Systematic reviews (ROBIS) which evaluates RoB in the review most specifically concerned with disease diagnosis and prognosis.[30] ROBIS can be accessed at http://www.bristol.ac.uk/population-health-sciences/projects/robis/. Other tools are available and require greater review regarding their utility in the conduct and reporting of systematic reviews and meta-analyses.

SUMMARY

Evidence synthesis is a complex approach to research that can be a powerful tool when used correctly. The hierarchy of this field is based upon the concepts of transparency and reproducibility starting with the narrative review and ending with the meta-analysis. This article was meant to provide an overview of the subject as well as the foundations of the different designs within evidence synthesis. Evidence synthesis research involves the rigorous and comprehensive examination of existing research literature on a particular topic. Its aim is to synthesize and analyze the available evidence from multiple peer-reviewed sources to draw meaningful conclusions and inform decision-making. The preceding passage has outlined the methodology to identify, select, appraise, and analyze the pertinent studies. Researchers must systematically search databases, screen articles based on predefined criteria, assess the quality and RoB of the included studies, and extract relevant data. This predetermined process optimizes the objectivity of reviewed evidence. The results of evidence synthesis research provide a comprehensive summary of the current understanding of a particular topic. The combination of data from multiple studies allows researchers to identify patterns, trends, and inconsistencies across the literature. This process minimizes the RoB, increases statistical power, and provides more robust conclusions than individual study results. Well-executed evidence synthesis research informs both policy-making and clinical decision-making in a way that resonates for years.

DISCLOSURE

The authors and contributors of this article declare that they have no financial conflicts of interest related to the content presented. The information reported is derived from individual expertise in concert with comprehensive review of reliable sources as detailed in the References section.

REFERENCES

1. Munn Z, Peters MDJ, Stern C, et al. Systematic review or scoping review? Guidance for authors when choosing between a systematic or scoping review approach. BMC Med Res Methodol 2018;18(1):143.
2. Arksey H, O'Malley L. Scoping studies: towards a methodological framework. Int J Soc Res Methodol 2005;8(1):19–32.
3. Medical College of Wisconsin. Evidence Based Medicine: PICO. Medical College of Wisconsin Libraries. Accessed June 12, 2023. https://mcw.libguides.com/EBM/PICO.
4. University of Melbourne. Systematic Reviews for Health Sciences and Medicine: Inclusion and exclusion criteria. University of Melbourne Library. Accessed June 12, 2023. https://unimelb.libguides.com/sysrev/inclusion-exclusion-criteria.
5. University of Texas. Systematic Reviews: Inclusion and Exclusion Criteria. University of Texas Library. Accessed June 12, 2023. https://libguides.sph.uth.tmc.edu/SystematicReviews/InclusionAndExclusion.
6. Moher D, Pham B, Lawson ML, et al. The inclusion of reports of randomised trials published in languages other than English in systematic reviews. Health Technol Assess 2003;7(41):1–90.
7. Morrison A, Polisena J, Husereau D, et al. The effect of English-language restriction on systematic review-based meta-analyses: a systematic review of empirical studies. Int J Technol Assess Health Care 2012;28(2):138–44.
8. Elsevier. What is Web of Science and how does it work? Elsevier. Accessed June 12, 2023. https://service.elsevier.com/app/answers/detail/a_id/34311/supporthub/publishing/.
9. University of Liverpool. What is Ovid and how do I access and use it? University Of Liverpool Library. Accessed June 12, 2023. https://libanswers.liverpool.ac.uk/faq/133906.
10. University of Tasmania. Systematic Reviews for Health: Develop Search Terms. University of Tasmania Library. Accessed June 12, 2023. https://utas.libguides.com/SystematicReviews/ControlledVocabularyTerms.
11. Higgins J, Chandler J, Cumpston M, Li T, Page M, Welch V, eds Cochraine Handbook for Systematic Review of Interventions. 6.3.; 2022. www.training.cochrane.org/handbook.
12. Kwon Y, Lemieux M, McTavish J, et al. Identifying and removing duplicate records from systematic review searches. J Med Libr Assoc 2015;103(4):184–8.
13. Gøtzsche PC, Hróbjartsson A, Maric K, et al. Data extraction errors in meta-analyses that use standardized mean differences. JAMA 2007;298(4):430–7.
14. WebPlotDigitizer. WebPlot Digitizer. Available at: https://apps.automeris.io/wpd/. Accessed June 12, 2023.
15. Hedin RJ, Umberham BA, Detweiler BN, et al. Publication bias and nonreporting found in majority of systematic reviews and meta-analyses in anesthesiology journals. Anesth Analg 2016;123(4):1018–25.
16. Dalton JE, Bolen SD, Mascha EJ. Publication bias: the elephant in the review. Anesth Analg 2016;123(4):812–3.
17. Peters JL, Sutton AJ, Jones DR, et al. Contour-enhanced meta-analysis funnel plots help distinguish publication bias from other causes of asymmetry. J Clin Epidemiol 2008;61(10):991–6.
18. Jadad AR, Moore RA, Carroll D, et al. Assessing the quality of reports of randomized clinical trials: is blinding necessary? Control Clin Trials 1996;17(1):1–12.

19. Schulz KF, Altman DG, Moher D, CONSORT Group. CONSORT 2010 statement: updated guidelines for reporting parallel group randomised trials. BMJ 2010;340: c332.
20. Higgins JPT, Altman DG, Gøtzsche PC, et al. The Cochrane Collaboration's tool for assessing risk of bias in randomised trials. BMJ 2011;343:d5928.
21. Page MJ, McKenzie JE, Bossuyt PM, et al. The PRISMA 2020 statement: an updated guideline for reporting systematic reviews. BMJ 2021;372:n71.
22. Oxford Reference. Overview: metameter. Oxford Dictionary of Biochemistry and Molecular Biology. doi:10.1093/oi/authority.20110803100153971.
23. Huedo-Medina TB, Sánchez-Meca J, Marín-Martínez F, et al. Assessing heterogeneity in meta-analysis: Q statistic or I^2 index? Psychol Methods 2006;11(2): 193–206.
24. Parlett-Pelleriti C. What the **** is a Q Statistic. Available at:https://cmparlettpelleriti.github.io/QStatistic.html. Accessed June 12, 2023.
25. von Hippel PT. The heterogeneity statistic I2 can be biased in small meta-analyses. BMC Med Res Methodol 2015;15(1):35.
26. Moher D, Liberati A, Tetzlaff J, et al, PRISMA Group. Preferred reporting items for systematic reviews and meta-analyses: the PRISMA statement. Ann Intern Med 2009;151(4):264–9.
27. Brooke BS, Schwartz TA, Pawlik TM. MOOSE reporting guidelines for meta-analyses of observational studies. JAMA Surg 2021;156(8):787–8.
28. Stroup DF, Berlin JA, Morton SC, et al. Meta-analysis of observational studies in epidemiology: a proposal for reporting. Meta-analysis of Observational Studies in Epidemiology (MOOSE) group. JAMA 2000;283(15):2008–12.
29. Shea BJ, Reeves BC, Wells G, et al. Amstar 2: a critical appraisal tool for systematic reviews that Include randomised or non-randomised studies of healthcare interventions, or both. BMJ 2017;358:j4008.
30. Whiting P, Savović J, Higgins JPT, et al. ROBIS: a new tool to assess risk of bias in systematic reviews was developed. J Clin Epidemiol 2016;69:225–34.

A Primer on Cost-Effectiveness Analysis

Rachel H. Albright, DPM, MPH[a],*, Adam E. Fleischer, DPM, MPH[b,c]

KEYWORDS

- Cost-effectiveness analysis • Cost analysis • Health economics

KEY POINTS

- Cost-effectiveness analyses (CEAs) are used to aid in health-care decisions.
- A formal CEA can be easily differentiated from a crude cost analysis by the inclusion of an incremental cost-effectiveness ratio term (a ratio of the costs and effectiveness of 2 competing strategies).
- Considering trade-offs and multiple perspectives are key components to a CEA.
- Results of a CEA are interpreted in relative terms (that is—strategy A is cost-effective in comparison to strategy B for condition X). It is not appropriate to say strategy A is cost-effective without specifying the comparing strategy.
- Uncertainty surrounding CEA is managed via sensitivity and probabilistic sensitivity analysis.

INTRODUCTION

The term *cost analysis* is a broad term to describe several different financial analyses that exist, all with the same goal—which is to help the user make more informed, and in many cases, better decisions. Cost analyses are used in many different fields besides health care. For example, the finance and business sectors use cost analysis (typically in the form of cost–benefit analyses or cost utility analyses) to evaluate future investments and determine which are more likely to bring forth the highest revenue with the least amount of risk. In health care, we are performing a similar analysis but our goals and objectives differ from profit optimization. The goals and objectives in health care are to prevent poor outcomes, prevent disease occurrence, and/or stifle the disease process, all with the intention of improving quality of life.[1,2] The common cost analysis used in health care is cost-effectiveness analysis (CEA). Decision analyses are also a helpful tool that enables the user to make more informed health-care

a Depatment of Surgery, Podiatry, Foot & Ankle Surgery, Stamford Health Medical Group, 800 Post Road, Suite 302, Darien, CT 06820, USA; b Weil Foot & Ankle Institute, 1660 Feehanville Drive, Suite 100, Mount Prospect, IL 60056, USA; c Rosalind Franklin University of Medicine & Science, 3333 Green Bay Road, North Chicago, IL 60064, USA
* Corresponding author. 800 Post Road, Suite 302, Darien, CT 06820.
E-mail address: albrightrh@gmail.com

Clin Podiatr Med Surg 41 (2024) 313–321
https://doi.org/10.1016/j.cpm.2023.07.006
0891-8422/24/© 2023 Elsevier Inc. All rights reserved.

podiatric.theclinics.com

decisions but does not routinely incorporate cost data. Both decision analysis and CEA come under the umbrella of "health economics." For the purposes of this article, we will focus solely on CEA.

BACKGROUND

It is important to understand the term *health economics* and appreciate the foundational purpose of this area of study. Health economics (in simple terms) is essentially trying to achieve better health-care decision-making by analyzing how resources are being allocated in the health-care system. This stems from the understanding that resources are limited, and decisions need to be made to determine how to use them.[3,4] Questions answered by health economics may include the following:

- How is health care valued in a particular system?
- What influences demand for health care?
- What are the alternative ways we can supply and deliver health care?
- How can we maximize our outcomes with the resources we currently have?
- How should resources should be allocated and what is a fair way to allocate the resources?
- Where are we currently using our money in health care and is this an effective way to be using it?

The challenge in health-care economics is the realization that medical decision-making is a complex process. There are very few instances in health care that presents a patient with a simple decision—where if given all the knowledge at hand, will still render a very simple answer. Medical decisions do not always include the amount of transparency that we need to make an informed decision. For example, there are rarely only 2 outcomes possible, and the outcomes presented are not always certain to occur. When we consider the consequences (or side effects) of treatment, some of these consequences will be immediate while others may occur over time. Some outcomes will have financial costs, emotional costs, and psychological costs that are difficult to determine and measure. Some outcomes/side effects of treatment might range from a very minor inconvenience to severe disability, or even death. To add to the complexity, medical decisions are not often made by a single person but may involve family members, friends, and other stakeholders (eg, the health-care system). All these things considered, there is still the question of how much money is worth spending to achieve a certain outcome and what level of certainty is required to take this risk.

What Is Cost-Effectiveness Analysis?

A CEA is a type of health economics model that uses a systematic approach to simplify the complexities that exist in health-care decision-making. This approach involves (1) identifying a problem, (2) identifying the available, competing treatment strategies, (3) identifying the consequences and trade-offs of the treatment strategies, (4) evaluating the evidence (eg, costs and events), (5) finding a simplified way to measure health and finally, and (6) determining the value of each strategy. Health is typically depicted as a health utility (ie, a way to describe a current state of health) which, when accumulated, corresponds to life years, quality-adjusted life years (QALYs), or disability adjusted life years (DALYs). Life years have been met with some criticism. It is recognized that a longer life is not necessarily a better life, especially if some of the years lived, are lived in disability and are of poor quality. QALYs have therefore been the preferred adopted measure of health in CEAs. QALYs give more value to the years lived in good health and less value to years lived in poor health. DALYs are typically used in underdeveloped countries and would not be an appropriate variable for CEAs depicting the US population or other developed countries. A computer-simulated model is then used to evaluate the problem considering the available data. The combination of the costs ($, USD) and effectiveness (ie, QALYs) of 2 treatment strategies are combined to form the incremental cost-effectiveness ratio (ie, ICER, the main outcome measure).

A CEA aids in medical decision-making by considering both the costs and the outcomes of at least 2 competing strategies. This is a distinct difference to a crude cost analysis, which is commonly found in the literature yet is often inappropriately interpreted to yield cost-effectiveness data. There are several distinct differences between the crude cost analysis and the CEA (**Table 1**). One evident difference that makes a CEA easy to identify is the outcome measure used. All CEAs are going to use a variable that integrates both costs and outcomes, combining 2 competing strategies into one, meaningful value-based term. This value-based term is a ratio of the 2 strategies and is called the ICER. A crude cost analysis, however, will examine the cost of strategy A versus the cost of strategy B, and then, separately look at the outcomes of strategy A versus the outcomes of strategy B. A crude cost analysis does not attempt to integrate costs and outcomes together. The cost and the outcomes that are produced by a crude cost analysis are absolute values and not relative values. It is important for the reader to understand that an absolute value will have limited meaning in the context of medical decision-making because of the high complexity of the decisions being made. For example, knowing the cost of strategy A is US$100,000 and the cost of strategy B is US$50,000 has limited meaning because this comparison alone does not consider the other important factors used to make real-life decisions. The risks of each of these strategies, the probability of complications of the strategy, the probability of side effects produced by the strategies, and the influence of these strategies on the person that might be receiving them are all important aspects of decision-making. Therefore, saying that strategy B costs half the amount of strategy A without placing it into the context of the different trade-offs that come with each strategy has very little meaning in real-world medical decision-making and should be discouraged. This is the same for comparing outcomes where an author can conclude that strategy A has a better outcome than strategy B but does not consider how these outcomes might be perceived by different groups of people, in different time periods, and at different cost points. It is therefore inappropriate for a crude cost analysis to make a conclusion that a strategy is "cost-effective." This error is commonly made in the medical literature and journal editors should be mindful of this error and encourage authors to avoid using the term "cost-effective" to describe a strategy that has not undergone a formal CEA.

Are There Bad Questions to Ask of a Cost-Effectiveness Analysis?

A CEA may not always be necessary to help physicians and decision makers determine the best course of action. For example, in a situation where we know that strategy A is more effective compared with strategy B, and in addition, we also know that strategy A is cheaper than strategy B, then a CEA would not be needed. A reader would already have an understanding that strategy A is the recommended strategy for treating the condition in question. Analysis is only needed when there is conflicting evidence, where a more expensive strategy has an unknown outcome and/or which strategy might be cheaper in certain clinical scenarios. This is commonly seen in oncology research. Many of the treatment strategies used for cancer treatment are expensive yet if they can render a higher quality of life to the person, or prolong years

Table 1
Are there bad questions to ask of a cost-effectiveness analysis?

	Crude Cost Analysis	CEA
Purpose	• Provides data for future CEA • Hypothesis generating	Aid in medical decision-making for complex clinical scenarios
Outcome assessed	Varies	• Integrates costs and outcomes into one value • Primary outcome is an ICER
Design	• Multiple study types (typically retrospective and prospective cohorts)	Computer simulation model
Analysis	Varies according to design	• Simple CEA • Markov model • Microsimulation
Result interpretation	• Strategy A is more *effective* than strategy B for the treatment of condition X • Strategy A is more *expensive* than strategy B for the treatment of condition X • Results are not typically considered in the context of multiple viewpoints	• Results are interpreted in the context of multiple viewpoints • Results are relative to other strategy considered • Strategy A is cost-effective in comparison to strategy B for the treatment of condition X
Nuances	• No trade-offs considered • Cannot give insight into whether a strategy offers "value"	• Considers trade-offs • Health must be simplified into an easier yet meaningful term (such as quality of life, life years, years in disability)

of life in a person, then the increased cost might be justified to warrant using that strategy. A CEA can aid a physician in making this determination.

Key Concepts in Cost-Effectiveness Analysis

The term *trade-off* is used routinely in health economics, and it represents the risks and benefits of the decision at hand. Trade-offs are an essential component to CEA. It is vitally important that health-care analyses identify relevant trade-offs and capture these within the health-care model. For example, if looking at a treatment strategy that involves surgical intervention, a common trade-off to consider is weighing any immediate risks that are involved concerning the procedure itself versus the improved long-term prognosis or quality of life that could be achieved by undergoing the procedure. Oftentimes, the consequence of the procedure is not one single outcome. There are often several consequences that one might consider. Additionally, each person has a different opinion on which of these consequences will have a greater impact on his/her personal life.

A cost-effectiveness model is reframed several times to integrate the perspectives of many different viewpoints. For example, at minimum, most health economic models consider the viewpoint of the health-care system. The health-care system's perspective considers the probability of a bad outcome and the cost associated with that outcome, the likelihood of achieving a good outcome, and what quality of life the person may achieve for a certain cost. Because the health-care system must be willing to pay for the treatment options, this perspective is an important one. However, experts in health economics have recognized that the viewpoint of the patient and/or the social/societal viewpoint is also an important aspect of health-care modeling.[8] The societal viewpoint considers factors such as lost wages, time off work, transportation to outpatient appointments, and emotional or psychological losses that the patient might experience including possible stigmas surrounding certain health-care conditions.[3] For example, the physician holds the understanding regarding the possible range of outcomes a person may experience following treatment. He/she may also have an understanding of the likelihood of each outcome. However, the patient holds the understanding of their personal preferences, their anxieties, and their wants and needs. Both of these assessments will play a role in good decision-making.

Reframing the health-care model from multiple perspectives can often yield different results and may lead the patient to a different decision. The most comprehensive models will therefore consider multiple perspectives. With all these difference considerations, it is important for health-care models to not lose sight of the main objective, which is to cure, stifle, or prevent disease and improve quality of life. In some circumstances, the prevention or cure of disease may be the goal but in other instances, it might be slowing the disease process. Regardless of the specific goal, a good health-care model will consider every relevant treatment regimen that is currently being used for a disease. There are many instances where watchful waiting is a reasonable alternative, and this should be considered as a treatment strategy when appropriate.

Capturing Costs

There are often questions regarding how one can capture the totality of costs raising issue with how imprecise cost estimates are. It is important to understand that it is not required to capture the totality of cost in order to help make a better medical decision. There are strict guidelines that exist to assist a researcher in performing a meaningful CEA.[4,5] One requirement of a CEA is to ensure that multiple perspectives or viewpoints are considered (as noted above). Each perspective will incorporate and represent a different list of important costs that are associated with each treatment strategy.

Common viewpoints, as mentioned earlier, are the health-care perspective and the social/societal perspective. The health-care perspective is going to be concerned with costs associated with the treatment strategy itself and include both direct and indirect costs. Direct costs include the cost of the treatment strategy, the cost of postoperative care, the cost of complications and side effects, physician costs, and so forth. Indirect costs associated with the health-care perspective include new disease states that may occur long term, durable medical equipment needed in the future, imaging studies, and so forth. The societal perspective is more difficult to incorporate and considers opportunity costs, productivity and/or time costs (time off work, transportation, outpatient appointments and tests), and community preferences.[5] CEAs should aim to include the societal perspective but given the difficulty in obtaining these values, it is not always incorporated. A CEA performed as a secondary analysis from a randomized controlled trial (RCT) has a unique opportunity to obtain the societal perspective and often render the most robust CEAs found in the literature. It would be considered an unfortunate oversight for a CEA to not consider the societal perspective if there is access to RCT data and would stifle a CEA's influence by not taking advantage of this privilege that others find difficult to obtain.

When a researcher is not afforded the opportunity to use data from a randomized trial, using the available medical literature is a reasonable second option. The authors should attempt a comprehensive, thorough review of the medical literature to obtain applicable data and may pool the data using meta-analysis to form estimates surrounding possible trade-offs. An example of this can be found in our previous study where we examine surgical treatment options for Charcot arthropathy using available literature.[6]

Managing Uncertainty

Sensitivity analysis is an essential component to a CEA. A sensitivity analysis is a way for the researcher to address the issues of uncertainty surrounding the model. It allows the researcher to vary the costs and probabilities of events to see if this will change the results. Sensitivity analysis can change one variable at a time (one-way sensitivity) or multiple variables (multiway sensitivity) at the same time. Researchers can then offer the reader assured confidence that the model is accurate in several clinical scenarios or, offer words of caution if the model shows volatility in certain clinical scenarios. A probabilistic analysis is a sensitivity analysis that uses a wide, but relevant, distribution of data to form different clinical scenarios. For example, ranging the mean of a variable 10 different times will offer 10 scenarios for determining which treatment is the best option. If the same treatment strategy is preferred 8 out of 10 times, this gives the reader some confidence that this variable is not greatly affecting the results of the model—that is—about 80% of time, the results are the same regardless of changes to the variable. In a probabilistic analysis, however, a distribution of data is used to test variables. These distributions can be assigned to multiple variables at the same time, producing tens of thousands of scenarios for consideration. The researcher has the ability to run the model hundreds of thousands of times using these distributions of data. If the model shows a strategy is preferred 80% of the time after being run tens of thousands of times in different scenarios, this offers even more confidence to the reader. Additionally, a probabilistic analysis can be used to formulate confidence intervals around the final model's mean. This type of analysis is welcomed and, in many ways, expected for a more comprehensive CEA. To this end, a probabilistic analysis should always be attempted. Similar to the types of statistical analyses that most researchers in the United States are more comfortable with, such as regression analysis, a probabilistic analysis will produce a confidence interval. These confidence intervals can often have even more certainty surrounding them than a typical regression analysis and are typically 97.5% confidence intervals instead of the typical 95% confidence intervals. The power of these sensitivity analyses suggest that a CEA does not present any additional uncertainty compared with any other statistical model that researchers are comfortable doing. When sensitivity and probabilistic sensitivity analysis are performed properly, there is little reason to think that the model has additional uncertainty surrounding it compared with another statistical model. It can be argued that the same skepticism surrounding uncertainty in CEA should be equally given to randomized control trials and other accepted methods that have limitations in the number of variables considered, typically do not consider multiple perspectives, and do not measure the trade-offs that exist in real-life decisions. CEA will continue to be subject to criticism while the technique is unfamiliar.

Interpretation of Cost-Effectiveness Analysis Results

The interpretation of a CEA can be difficult. When considering publication, interpretation will be easier when authors are transparent about all aspects of the model, including providing the base case scenarios for costs and events, how quality of life was measured, and health utilities. The decision tree should be shared when it is reasonable to do so (an example of this can be found in the reference).[7] When the decision tree cannot be shared (eg, in instances where the tree is too complex to be visually depicted), then a state transition diagram with a description of possible events should be supplied. Including these aspects of the model helps the reader to determine if the model represents an accurate and meaningful clinical scenario. The closer the model mimics real-life scenarios, the more applicable the analysis and results will be to the reader. It is important to understand that a CEA should only be interpreted in terms of relative value. For example, it would be inappropriate to say that, "Strategy A is a cost-effective strategy for Condition X." CEAs identify strategies that are cost-effective only in comparison to another reasonable, competing strategy. A more appropriate way to interpret the results would be "Strategy A is a cost-effective strategy in comparison to strategy B for the treatment of condition X." When more than 2 strategies are analyzed, each strategy is compared with the next cheaper option (not the overall cheapest option). The ICER determines if a strategy is cost-effective in comparison to another option. If the ICER falls below a set willingness-to-pay, then the strategy is considered cost-effective in comparison to the next cheaper option. In the United States, the willingness-to-pay ranges anywhere from US$50,000 to US$150,000 and represents the amount of money the health-care system is willing to pay to gain one additional quality adjusted life year. However, many authors have argued against these arbitrary figures and have instead recommended a threshold that is based on a country's gross domestic product.[8] It is important to note that the ICER alone cannot determine whether the benefit of an intervention is worth the cost. Cost-effectiveness is always a relative term that reflects the price of additional units of benefit. Results may additionally be interpreted from multiple perspectives where different viewpoints may yield different preferred strategies.

SUMMARY

CEAs are models that take a large sum of data to simplify a decision-making process. These can be used by an individual provider, policymakers, or insurance companies to decide which treatment strategies are going to be funded for their beneficiaries. It is important to note that 10 years from now, the truth might change as new evidence becomes available, more beliefs are considered, and more groups of people share their stories. Therefore, CEAs should probably be revisited and repeated when new evidence becomes available or when a significant amount of time passes.

Although some criticize CEA as being insufficient for truly making a profound healthcare decision, there is rarely an instance in life where we have all the information we need to make the best decision possible. We can only use the information at hand to make the best decision we can. There is uncertainty that surrounds almost every decision that we make but if we can become better at mitigating and communicating that uncertainty, then better health decisions can be made. When a CEA is performed appropriately, comprehensively, ethically, and keeping the objective of health care at the forefront, there is no question that a CEA is an invaluable model for aiding in better decision-making.

CLINICS CARE POINTS

- CEAs are used to aid in health-care decisions.
- A formal CEA can be easily differentiated from a crude cost analysis by the inclusion of an ICER term (a ratio of the costs and effectiveness of 2 competing strategies).
- Considering trade-offs and multiple perspectives are key components to a CEA.
- Results of a CEA are interpreted in relative terms (that is—Strategy A is cost-effective in comparison to strategy B for condition X). It is not appropriate to say strategy A is cost-effective without specifying the comparing strategy.
- Uncertainty surrounding CEA is managed via sensitivity and probabilistic sensitivity analysis.

DISCLOSURE

The authors have nothing to disclose.

ACKNOWLEDGEMENTS

** This article draws heavily on concepts presented in (Neumann P, Sanders, G., Russell, L., Siegel, J., Ganiats, T. *Cost-Effectiveness in Health and Medicine.* 2nd Edition ed. New York, New York: Oxford University Press; 2017.[7]) and (Hunink M, Weinstein, M., Wittenberg, E., Drummond, M., Pliskin, J., Wong, J., Glasziou, P. *Decision Making in Health and Medicine: Integrating Evidence and Values.* 2nd Edition ed. Cambridge, United Kingdom: Cambridge University Press; 2016.[8])

REFERENCES

1. Neumann P, Sanders G, Russell L, et al. *Cost-Effectiveness in Health and medicine.* 2nd edition. New York, New York: Oxford University Press; 2017.
2. Hunink M, Weinstein M, Wittenberg E, et al. Decision making in health and medicine: integrating evidence and values. Cambridge, United Kingdom: Cambridge University Press; 2016.
3. Drummond MF, Jefferson TO. Guidelines for authors and peer reviewers of economic submissions to the BMJ. The BMJ Economic Evaluation Working Party. BMJ 1996;313(7052):275–83.
4. Husereau D, Drummond M, Petrou S, et al. Consolidated health economic evaluation reporting standards (CHEERS) statement. BMJ Br Med J (Clin Res Ed) 2013;346:f1049.

5. Garrison LP, Mansley EC, Abbott TA, et al. Good research practices for measuring drug costs in cost-effectiveness analyses: a societal perspective: the ispor drug cost task force report—Part II. Value Health 2010;13(1):8–13.
6. Albright RH, Joseph RM, Wukich DK, et al. Is reconstruction of unstable midfoot Charcot neuroarthropathy cost effective from a US payer's perspective? Clin Orthop Relat Res 2020;478(12):2869–88.
7. Albright RH, Waverly BJ, Klein E, et al. Percutaneous kirschner wire versus commercial implant for hammertoe repair: a cost-effectiveness analysis. J Foot Ankle Surg 2018;57(2):332–8.
8. Yanovskiy M, Levy ON, Shaki YY, et al. Cost-effectiveness threshold for healthcare: justification and quantification. Inquiry 2022;59. 469580221081438.

Unique Challenges in Diabetic Foot Science

Craig Verdin, DPM, Caitlin Zarick, DPM, John Steinberg, DPM*

KEYWORDS

- Heterogeneity • Multifactorial • Wound closure and wound healing
- Mortality and morbidity • Major amputation • Minor amputation
- Ambulation and function

KEY POINTS

- Diabetes is a complex condition that we are only beginning to understand. As a result, its associated complications demonstrate significant heterogeneity in their presentation and progression.
- When podiatric intervention is required, the definition of success has evolved during the course of time, and there is increasingly a lack of consensus on what end goals should be targeted.
- Managing expectations on outcomes relating to closure, function, prevention of major amputation, and long-term outcomes should be considered to ensure better outcomes with less morbidity.

INTRODUCTION

Within the past 30 years, there has been a rapid influx of information pertaining to the diabetic foot (DF) coming from numerous directions and sources. With this rapid growth in the knowledge base of DF literature, it can be difficult for treating clinicians to process and properly use this volume of data. This article discusses the current state of the DF literature and the unique challenges it presents to clinicians with its associated increase in knowledge on their derivations, complications, and interventions. Further, we attempt to provide tips on how to navigate and criticize the current literature to encourage and maximize positive outcomes in this challenging patient population.

Diabetes is a systemic condition that has a widespread and multiorgan influence across the body. Given the vast interconnectedness of the human body, the literature has ample evidence of the global effect diabetes has on the human body. For the foot and ankle clinician who is focused on the complications of the lower extremity, this can make evidence-based care difficult and often unpredictable in this complex patient

Department of Plastic Surgery, MedStar Georgetown University Hospital, 3800 Reservoir Road NW, Washington DC 20007, USA
* Corresponding author.
E-mail address: steinberg@usa.net

Clin Podiatr Med Surg 41 (2024) 323–331
https://doi.org/10.1016/j.cpm.2023.08.003
0891-8422/24/© 2023 Elsevier Inc. All rights reserved.

population. For this reason, within diabetic literature, there is a wide range of reported outcomes for podiatric interventions, which is more a reflection of the unpredictable nature of the disease and its complications. The objectives of this article is to (1) discuss the literature and the obstacles that many researchers face when attempting to produce meaningful and impactful research and (2) examine translational strategies for incorporating empirical findings into clinical practice.

OBSTACLES WITHIN THE LITERATURE

The DF literature has grown tremendously in the past several decades, with more than 6000 articles being dedicated to the DF.[1] Along with the growth of knowledge about the causative factors of diabetes and its complications, we have seen a rapid growth in the means of detection, management, and treatment. Despite the rapid growth of the DF literature and technologies, the inherent difficulties and obstacles of diabetes and its complications have presented continued challenges and obstacles that place patients at risk for increased rates of morbidity and mortality. In 2019, an article published by Geiss and colleagues evaluated the rates of amputation, major and minor, and found that during the timeframe that was evaluated (2010–2015), there seems to be an increase in amputations at every level.[2] Although it is not clear why this pattern of increase in amputation was observed, it can only be assumed that with the increasing prevalence of diabetes, this rate will continue.[3]

Diabetes is a heterogeneous disease, and diabetic researchers are only just beginning to understand the variations of the disease's presentation, progression, and outcomes, in so far that few mathematical models exist due its convoluted complexity.[4] In 2 independent studies by Dennis and Zaharia and colleagues, at least 5 unique clusters of diabetic subgroups were identified based on their presentation and progression.[5,6] Further, regarding complications, Apelqvist identified another 5 diabetic subgroup clusters, which further demonstrates the disease's complexity.[7] Given the well-documented complexity of the disease, it can only be inferred that this hampers the efforts of the foot and ankle clinician who is treating the downstream complications within the lower extremity. When looking at the DF literature, there is an extensive amount of heterogeneity regarding patient population, response to intervention, and long-term outcomes. Heterogeneity is not unique to the DF literature and is often viewed as a reflection of our lack of understanding of a condition. As in any field, heterogeneity is an intrinsic obstacle because with its increase, there is a proportional decrease in statistical power, which, in turn, produces less impactful data.[8] Further, within the diabetic literature, the presence of heterogeneity is often underassessed.[9,10] The multifactorial nature of the DF includes poorly defined or interminable variables such as glucose control, vascular status, degree of neuropathy, peak plantar pressures, previous interventions, and functional and ambulatory status. When considering these items, it is clear why heterogeneity exists within the DF literature in terms of detection, management, and treatment. Heterogeneity is inevitable and difficult to account for, and therefore, there exists 2 common and accepted statistical means of assessing heterogeneity: I^2 and tau. These 2 tools are commonly used in fields such as psychology where heterogenous populations with diverse presentations and treatments exist. I^2 is a percentage estimation that quantifies and correlates observed variability in effect size to real variations in effect size.[11] Simply put, the lower the I^2, the more differences can be attributed to sampling error and vice versa. Unfortunately, I^2 is not a sufficient means of assessing differences in effect sizes of smaller samples. Moreover, in the context of the DF literature, many studies, especially interventional studies, are smaller in size. This, in turn, inherently results in a high amount of heterogeneity. For this reason, I^2 may not be appropriate.[12] However, tau, which is the standard deviation of an observed effect size, has been proposed to be a more valuable means of assessing heterogeneity because it is not affected by sample size.[13] For this reason, the use of tau is best suited for the evaluation of heterogeneity in meta-analyses, which typically demonstrate a significant amount of variability concerning sample size of targeted studies. The use of means to quantify heterogeneity should be considered by DF researchers; however, a current review of the literature demonstrated a Cochrane Review article by Marti-Carvajal that evaluated the use of growth factors in DF ulcerations. In this study that identified 28 randomized controlled trials (RCTs) consisting of 2365 patients, there was a significant amount of expected heterogeneity across the targeted studies. Further, a meta-analysis was deemed not possible in 11 trials due to the heterogeneity in the assessment of wound healing, reporting, and issues with patient follow-up further demonstrating the amount of heterogeneity that is present even in well-constructed RCTs.[13]

Heterogeneity within the diabetic population is something that clinicians may never be able to avoid, especially considering the growing knowledge of the multifactorial and intrinsic complexity of diabetes pathophysiology. Because it has been proposed that increased heterogeneity is a reflection of the increased lack of understanding of a targeted condition or intervention, the targeted reduction of heterogeneity in targeted sample sizes implies (1) increased understanding of the disease/intervention and (2) increased value of the findings related to the targeted disease/intervention.[8] Although heterogeneity can be used to assess success within the DF literature, this raises the questions on whether homogeneity should be targeted. Within the DF literature, homogeneity is not a commonplace but, when present, its benefit can be valuable. Population homogeneity should be targeted when assessing interventions but its utility is not as meaningful when trying to draw conclusions about a larger population. An example in which homogeneity may limit the clinical usefulness of data is risk factor analysis. Even without heterogeneity and maximal homogeneity, there remains the significant issue of bias in research and clinical application of that research.

Bias within the DF literature is commonplace and is typically seen as problematic in terms of being able to provide reliable evidence for which clinical decision-making should be based on.[14,15] In another systematic review by Dayya and colleagues, even the literature assessing the efficacy and utility of debridement, which is often regarded as being the standard of care in diabetic foot ulcers (DFUs), is seen as being plagued with bias—in so far, that all 30 RCTs evaluated were characterized as having "unclear" or "high risk of bias" when assessing factors that can cause selection, performance, detection, attrition, and reporting bias.[16] Fortunately, for clinicians who are attempting to interpret the value of RCTs, there are numerous tools available to assess whether or not bias exists. The most commonly used tool is the criteria provided in the Cochrane Handbook for Systematic Reviews of Interventions, which addresses sequence generation, selective outcome reporting, incomplete outcome data, allocation concealment, blinding, and other factors.[17] For cohort studies and case-control studies, researchers can also use the Newcastle-Ottowa Quality Assessment forms.[18]

With the numerous methodical obstacles that can be found within the DF literature, this raises the questions on how to mitigate the effects of the numerous potentially confounding variables to produce meaningful results that can continue to encourage an increase in positive outcomes. It is critical when composing a study or assessing results to identify confounding variables and to understand how they might influence the findings. DF literature is filled with numerous risk factors that are either difficult to quantify or they exist on a spectrum along with the several types of interventions, means of assessing success, and differing end points. One means of mitigating and controlling the effects of these variables is through matching. Matched case control studies are commonplace within literature but not as plentiful within diabetic literature. Case-control matching allows for the creation of a risk-factor group or a comparable control group to serve as a comparison, which allows for increase delineation and identification of causal relationships with the more common variables that undergo matching being age, sex, and race. The strength of matching is it allows for isolation of causal relationships that may not have otherwise been exposed due to the presence of confounding variables. Research in the DF is filled with numerous potentially confounding variables that can produce dramatically different results.[19] One weakness of matching is the unintended introduction of bias, typically due to poor matching. Poor examples of matching typically involve the assumption that a variable is potentially confounding, thus eliminating its effect, regardless of whether it is a true confounder.[19] Properly performed matching within the DF literature could be very advantageous and would reduce the remarkably high rate of heterogeneity that was previously discussed. For example, risk factors for the development of a diabetic foot ulcer are commonplace within literature. The most common risk factors for DFU development are neuropathy, foot deformity, previous amputation, vasculopathy, and poor glycemic control.[20] If one were to perform a study that attempted to evaluate outcomes in a particular group, then it would be appropriate to match patients with diabetes with peripheral neuropathy with patients of the same, patients with diabetes without peripheral neuropathy with the same, and so forth. Although matching seems to be a simple solution to mitigate the inherent variability of the diabetic population, it is often time consuming, can be costly, and can be difficult for smaller volume researchers.[21] For this reason, regression techniques are more commonplace, especially when attempting to characterize treatment effect.[22] Despite these perceived difficulties, the benefits are worthwhile and could make findings more impactful and applicable.

OUTCOMES IN THE DIABETIC FOOT LITERATURE

Aside from the inherent difficulties of variability, heterogeneity, and numerous confounding variables, there remains the challenge of extrapolation of research results and applying them to clinical practice. Within the DF literature, there are numerous endpoints for which clinicians may consider to be a "success." The results are numerous in their utility and assessment. Common end points within the literature are typically related to closure, wound healing rates, amputation rates, durability of intervention, functional and ambulatory outcomes, mortality, recurrence, and so forth. Although all of these should certainly be considered and targeted when applicable, their weighted value in the long-term success of clinical outcomes is fairly reader dependent. The goal of any limb preservation surgeon or wound clinician is the closure and healing of an open wound or ulceration. In turn, closure prevents adverse effects associated with DFUs such as infection, amputation, and mortality. Although the end goal remains the same for all clinicians, the literature is varied in the type of closure, evaluation, size, and type of studies, and even the definition and calculation of wound healing rates.[23–30] Even further, there are numerous examples of ancillary modalities that are often used as an adjunct to healing, which often involve the use of complex biologics, skin substitutes, hyperbaric oxygen therapy, and negative pressure wound therapy (NPWT). Closure can be obtained through 3 means: primary, delayed, or secondary. Primary closure can be performed by using native residual tissue, microsurgical techniques, or orthoplastic means.[31] Recently, orthoplastic and microsurgical closures have been increasingly advocated as a valuable means of seeking closure in traumatic wounds and are being used within diabetic limb salvage.[32] These options, however, are typically only available in resource-enriched regions, which many foot and ankle clinicians might not have ready access to.[33] Secondary closure is often performed through means of grafting, use of NPWT, or other ancillary methods. The indications for secondary closure are numerous but are often preceded by a wound that may not be appropriate for primary closure due to lack of native skin for closure or inability to undergo advanced soft tissue coverage procedures. Unfortunately, the literature is not replete in terms of comparing whether primary closure or delayed primary closure as compared with secondary closure results in improved outcomes. The literature that does exist demonstrates that all means of closure are equivalent in the long term. In a study by Ahmed and colleagues in 2016, 160 patients with diabetes and neuropathy with a DFU were evaluated to compare whether primary closure is superior to secondary closure to heal a DFU.[34] It was found that primary closure did result in quicker rates of closure and reduction of dressing changes but within this study, there is no mention of follow-up after healing. In another study by Garcia-Morales and colleagues, primary closure was evaluated against secondary closure in patients who previously had osteomyelitis.[35] Again, in this study it was found that primary closure results in shorter healing times but, again, no description of the long-term durability of the means of closure. In the most significant of studies, in 2006, Berceli and colleagues performed a study to evaluate the benefits of primary closure, staged closure, and open amputations.[36] Although the benefits of primary closure and staged closure result in quicker healing times and reduction of reinfection rates, the long-term benefits of primary closure were lost at 36 months, which raises questions on the longevity and durability of amputations. These studies demonstrate the significant difference in the literature in regards to the definition of "closure" and "healing" and that critical readers should pay close attention to these when evaluating research and applying it to their practice.

Historically, the goal of limb salvage is to preserve length and prevent major lower extremity amputation; however, recent literature has focused on the functional aspect of limb salvage.[37] Although, in principle, length preservation equates to increased ambulation rates, the functional consequences are underrecognized. In an article by Roukis and colleagues, it was found that up to 76% of patients who underwent a transmetatarsal amputation may have some form of residual deformity, with a high percentage of patients requiring amputation reconstruction.[38] It is well documented that the more progressive levels of pedal amputations are fraught with complications, which may be related to the inherent dysfunction that is associated with the loss of tendinous insertions and osseous length; however, a well-reconstructed amputation has been shown to have predictable rate of ambulation preservation as compared with transtibial amputations.[39,40] In turn, although pedal length may be preserved, it does not imply function is preserved. For this reason, Attinger and colleagues has advocated that a below the knee amputation (BKA) is more functional than poorly reconstructed and less-functional pedal amputation constructs.[41] Although BKAs are not immune from complications, the use of a well-constructed prosthesis is more attainable with a BKA as opposed to a several shortened partial foot amputation constructs, which, in turn, allow the patient to return to a targeted level of ambulation. The end point of many studies within the DF literature is a BKA or other major extremity amputation.[42] Unfortunately, many studies perceive the progression to a major lower extremity amputation (LEA) as a failure of therapy; however, not all patients that progress to a major LEA should be considered a failure, especially if the BKA results in them resuming ambulation.

Another commonly assessed end point in the DF literature is mortality.[43,44] The most common means of assessing mortality within the current literature is 30-day mortality and 1-year, 3-year, and 5-year mortalities.[45] The 30-day mortality is an important measure because it reflects institutional practices and is largely a performance measure.[46] Diabetics who undergo interventions that require hospitalization often have a significant number of comorbidities that place them at increased risk for morbidity and mortality.[47] Long-term mortality is a bit more convoluted and can be influenced by comorbidities and limb loss.[48] Mortality data is valuable because it allows clinicians to compare interventions to justify their use. A common example of mortality data utilization is the use of long-term mortality data when assessing the value of certain levels of amputation. Recent literature has shown that patients who undergo major LEA often exhibit increased rates of long-term mortality relative to minor amputations.[44] It is not clear if these increased rates are related to the associated cardiovascular deconditioning that is seen in more proximal amputations or if patients who undergo major LEA are simply a more comorbid population.[49,50]

Given the various amounts of end points found within the DF literature, it can potentially be difficult for clinicians to translate available data into their clinical practice. Unfortunately, there is no "best" metric to assess diabetic interventions and the topic evolves over time. Metrics to assess outcomes in all aspects of medicine that were used 20 years ago would be considered archaic or outdated as clinicians gain a better understanding of disease and interventions. Within the diabetic foot, our understanding of the disease has progressed significantly in the past 20 years, and this will influence our views on how to treat its complications. Recent literature has begun to trend toward assessing outcomes from a functional perspective as well as assessing patient-reported outcomes measures, which may very well be the new norm as compared with previously used measures that may not necessarily quantify the actual effects of our interventions.[51]

SUMMARY

The public health impact of the DF is becoming more understood in recent years with increased attention, research, and targeted health programs. Our review seeks to point out some of the significant challenges that are growing along with this progress. We have continuing concerns about the literature and the way in which we interpret the care that should best be practiced. We applaud groups, such as the International Working Group on the Diabetic Foot, which work to evaluate the literature and produce guidelines that can serve to help all of us better understand the proper directions to take in this challenging field. We continue to balance an embrace of new technologies with a proper reserved approach toward utilization of resources and safeguarding of patient outcomes. We look forward to what the coming decades will bring to this fascinating and growing field of the diabetic lower extremity.

CLINICS CARE POINTS

- A growing quantity of literature on DF presents a significant challange and we must be critical of the published materials so that clinical practice is consistently guided by science.

ACKNOWLEDGMENT

None.

DISCLOSURE

John Steinberg is a consultant for Integra and Medline.

REFERENCES

1. Deng P, Shi H, Pan X, et al. Worldwide research trends on diabetic foot ulcers (2004-2020): suggestions for researchers. J Diabetes Res 2022;2022:7991031.
2. Geiss LS, Li Y, Hora I, et al. Resurgence of diabetes-related nontraumatic lower-extremity amputation in the young and middle-aged adult U.S. Population. Diabetes Care 2019;42(1):50–4.
3. Casciato DJ, Yancovitz S, Thompson J, et al. Diabetes-related major and minor amputation risk increased during the COVID-19 pandemic. J Am Podiatr Med Assoc 2020;3:20–224.
4. Ajmera I, Swat M, Laibe C, et al. The impact of mathematical modeling on the understanding of diabetes and related complications. CPT Pharmacometrics Syst Pharmacol 2013;2:e54.
5. Dennis JM, Shields BM, Henley WE, et al. Disease progression and treatment response in data-driven subgroups of type 2 diabetes compared with models based on simple clinical features: an analysis using clinical trial data. Lancet Diabetes Endocrinol 2019;7(6):442–51.
6. Zaharia OP, Strassburger K, Strom A, et al, German Diabetes Study Group. Risk of diabetes-associated diseases in subgroups of patients with recent-onset diabetes: a 5-year follow-up study. Lancet Diabetes Endocrinol 2019;7(9):684–94.
7. Aplqvist E, Storm P, Käräjämäki A, et al. Novel subgroups of adult-onset diabetes and their association with outcomes: a data-driven cluster analysis of six variables. Lancet Diabetes Endocrinol 2018;6(5):361–9.
8. Linden AH, Hönekopp J. Heterogeneity of research results: a new perspective from which to assess and promote progress in psychological science. Perspect Psychol Sci 2021;16(2):358–76.
9. Aytug ZG, Rothstein HR, Zhou W, et al. Revealed or concealed? Transparency of procedures, decisions, and judgment calls in meta-analyses. Organ Res Methods 2012;15(1):103–33.
10. Ioannidis JP. Interpretation of tests of heterogeneity and bias in meta-analysis. J Eval Clin Pract 2008;14(5):951–7.
11. Huedo-Medina TB, Sánchez-Meca J, Marín-Martínez F, et al. Assessing heterogeneity in meta-analysis: Q statistic or I^2 index? Psychol Methods 2006;11:193–206.
12. Borenstein M, Higgins JP, Hedges LV, et al. Basics of meta-analysis: I^2 is not an absolute measure of heterogeneity. Res Synth Methods 2017;8(1):5–18.
13. Martí-Carvajal AJ, Gluud C, Nicola S, et al. Growth factors for treating diabetic foot ulcers. Cochrane Database Syst Rev 2015;2015(10):CD008548.
14. van Erp S, Verhagen J, Grasman RP, et al. Estimates of between-study heterogeneity for 705 meta-analyses reported in *Psychological Bulletin* from 1990–2013. J Open Psychol Data 2017;5(1). Article 4.
15. Crawford F, Nicolson DJ, Amanna AE, et al. Reliability of the evidence to guide decision-making in foot ulcer prevention in diabetes: an overview of systematic reviews. BMC Med Res Methodol 2022;22(1):274.
16. Dayya D, O'Neill O, Habib N, et al. Debridement of diabetic foot ulcers: public health and clinical implications - a systematic review, meta-analysis, and meta-regression. BMJ Surg Interv Health Technol 2022;4(1):e000081.

17. Higgins JPT, Green S (editors). Cochrane Handbook for systematic reviews of interventions Version 5.1.0 (updated March 2011). The Cochrane Collaboration. Available at www.cochrane-handbook.org.
18. Wells GA, Shea B, O'Connell D, et al.The Newcastle-Ottawa Scale (NOS) for assessing the quality of nonrandomized studies in meta-analyses. http://www.ohri.ca/programs/clinical_epidemiology/oxford.asp. Accessed January 8th, 2023.
19. Strauss MB, Moon H, La S, et al. The incidence of confounding factors in patients with diabetes mellitus hospitalized for diabetic foot ulcers. Wounds 2016;28(8): 287–94.
20. Armstrong DG, Boulton AJM, Bus SA. Diabetic foot ulcers and their recurrence. N Engl J Med 2017;376(24):2367–75.
21. Cenzer I, Boscardin WJ, Berger K. Performance of matching methods in studies of rare diseases: a simulation study. Intractable Rare Dis Res 2020;9(2):79–88.
22. Deberneh HM, Kim I. Prediction of type 2 diabetes based on machine learning algorithm. Int J Environ Res Public Health 2021;18(6):3317.
23. Cukjati D, Reberšek S, Miklavčič D. A reliable method of determining wound healing rate. Med Biol Eng Comput 2001;39:263–71.
24. Arciero JC, Mi Q, Branca MF, et al. Continuum model of collective cell migration in wound healing and colony expansion. Biophys J 2011;100:535–43.
25. Gilman T. Wound outcomes: the utility of surface measures. Int J Low Extrem Wounds 2004;3:125–32.
26. Robson MC, Hill DP, Woodske ME, et al. Wound healing trajectories as predictors of effectiveness of therapeutic agents. Arch Surg 2000;135(7):773–7.
27. Sherratt JA, Murray JD. Mathematical analysis of a basic model for epidermal wound healing. J Math Biol 1991;29:389–404.
28. Sherratt JA, Murray JD. Epidermal wound healing: the clinical implications of a simple mathematical model. Cell Transplant 1992;1:365–71.
29. Tranquillo RT, Murray JD. Mechanistic model of wound contraction. J Surg Res 1993;55:233–47.
30. Wallenstein S, Brem H. Statistical analysis of wound-healing rates for pressure ulcers. Am J Surg 2004;188(1A suppl I):73–8.
31. Simman R, Abbas FT. Foot wounds and the reconstructive ladder. Plast Reconstr Surg Glob Open 2021;9(12):e3989.
32. Klifto KM, Azoury SC, Othman S, et al. The value of an orthoplastic approach to management of lower extremity trauma: systematic review and meta-analysis. Plast Reconstr Surg Glob Open 2021;9(3):e3494.
33. Fan KL, Singh T, Bekeny JC, et al. Use of flap salvage for lower extremity chronic wounds occurs most often in competitive hospital Markets. Plast Reconstr Surg Glob Open 2021;9(2):e3183.
34. Ahmed ME, Mohammed MS, Mahadi SI. Primary wound closure of diabetic foot ulcers by debridement and stitching. J Wound Care 2016;25(11):650–4.
35. García-Morales E, Lázaro-Martínez JL, Aragón-Sánchez J, et al. Surgical complications associated with primary closure in patients with diabetic foot osteomyelitis. Diabet Foot Ankle 2012;3. https://doi.org/10.3402/dfa.v3i0.19000.
36. Berceli SA, Brown JE, Irwin PB, et al. Clinical outcomes after closed, staged, and open forefoot amputations. J Vasc Surg 2006;44(2):347–51 [discussion: 352].
37. Dillon MP, Barker TM. Preservation of residual foot length in partial foot amputation: a biomechanical analysis. Foot Ankle Int 2006;27(2):110–6.
38. Roukis TS, Singh N, Andersen CA. Preserving functional capacity as opposed to tissue preservation in the diabetic patient: a single institution experience Foot. Ankle Spec 2010;3(4):177–83.

39. Kim PJ. Biomechanics of the diabetic foot: consideration in limb salvage. Adv Wound Care 2013;2(3):107–11.
40. Brown ML, Tang W, Patel A, et al. Partial foot amputation in patients with diabetic foot ulcers. Foot Ankle Int 2012;33(9):707–16.
41. Attinger CE, Brown BJ. Amputation and ambulation in diabetic patients: function is the goal. Diabetes Metab Res Rev 2012;28(Suppl 1):93–6.
42. Thorud JC, Jupiter DC, Lorenzana J, et al. Reoperation and reamputation after transmetatarsal amputation: a systematic review and meta-analysis. J Foot Ankle Surg 2016;55(5):1007–12.
43. Jupiter DC, Thorud JC, Buckley CJ, et al. The impact of foot ulceration and amputation on mortality in diabetic patients. I: from ulceration to death, a systematic review. Int Wound J 2016;13(5):892–903.
44. Thorud JC, Plemmons B, Buckley CJ, et al. Mortality after nontraumatic major amputation among patients with diabetes and peripheral vascular disease: a systematic review. J Foot Ankle Surg 2016;55(3):591–9.
45. Hirji S, McGurk S, Kiehm S, et al. Utility of 90-day mortality vs 30-day mortality as a quality metric for transcatheter and surgical aortic valve replacement outcomes. JAMA Cardiol 2020;5(2):156–65.
46. Panagiotou OA, Voorhies KR, Keohane LM, et al. Association of inclusion of medicare advantage patients in hospitals' risk-standardized readmission rates, performance, and penalty status. JAMA Netw Open 2021;4(2):e2037320.
47. Raghavan S, Vassy JL, Ho YL, et al. Diabetes mellitus-related all-cause and cardiovascular mortality in a National cohort of adults. J Am Heart Assoc 2019;8(4):e011295.
48. Vogel TR, Petroski GF, Kruse RL. Impact of amputation level and comorbidities on functional status of nursing home residents after lower extremity amputation. J Vasc Surg 2014;59(5):1323–13230.e1.
49. Pinzur MS, Gold J, Schwartz D, et al. Energy demands for walking in dysvascular amputees as related to the level of amputation. Orthopedics 1992;15(9):1033–6 [discussion: 1036-7].
50. Mundell BF, Luetmer MT, Kremers HM, et al. The risk of major cardiovascular events for adults with transfemoral amputation. J NeuroEng Rehabil 2018;15(Suppl 1):58.
51. Pérez-Panero AJ, Ruiz-Muñoz M, Fernández-Torres R, et al. Diabetic foot disease: a systematic literature review of patient-reported outcome measures. Qual Life Res 2021;30(12):3395–405.

Special Considerations in Podiatric Science
Translational Research, Cadavers, Gait Analysis, Dermatology, and Databases

Jarrett D. Cain, DPM[a], Tracey Vlahovic, DPM[b],
Andrew J. Meyr, DPM[c],*

KEYWORDS

- Benchtop • Mechanical testing • Force plate • Newton • Tinea • NSQIP

KEY POINTS

- Translational research involves the process of bringing basic science from the benchtop to interventional clinical application.
- Cadaveric methodologies generally involve either static or dynamic anatomic outcomes.
- Gait analysis and pressure measurement investigations might provide a more comprehensive and *in vivo* assessment of kinematic outcomes.
- The podiatric dermatology literature shares many outcomes with other dermatology literature, but critical readers should be aware of several specific inherent challenges.
- Database investigations are becoming more prevalent in the foot and ankle literature, and represent an opportunity for the scientific advancement of the profession.

KEY/ESSENTIAL HEADINGS
Translational Podiatric Science

Life expectancy is expected to rise to 85.9 years and 93.3 years for males and females, respectively, in the United States by 2050.[1] As the population ages, musculoskeletal conditions will become an increasing burden within the older population and on the health care system.[2] This places a demand across multiple specialties and fields to develop innovative treatments to address the rising number of patients affected by acute and chronic diseases. It also, however, creates an opportunity for clinicians

[a] Department of Orthopedic Surgery, University of Pittsburgh School of Medicine, University of Pittsburgh Physicians, 1515 Locust Street #350, Pittsburgh, PA 15219, USA; [b] Department of Medicine, Temple University School of Podiatric Medicine, 148 North 8th Street, Philadelphia, PA 19107, USA; [c] Department of Surgery, Temple University School of Podiatric Medicine, 148 North 8th Street, Philadelphia, PA 19107, USA
* Corresponding author.
E-mail address: ajmeyr@gmail.com

Clin Podiatr Med Surg 41 (2024) 333–341
https://doi.org/10.1016/j.cpm.2023.07.007

and scientists to gain a greater understanding of the diseases of the foot and ankle through translational research.

Translational research includes the process of applying discoveries initially generated in the laboratory and preclinical studies into the development of clinical trials and in-vivo investigations.[3] It also involves enhancing the adoption of best practices in the community including studying the cost-effectiveness of prevention-based and direct treatment interventions.[4] The translational research model is based on basic science, clinical application, and community health.[5] Basic science provides a fundamental understanding of diseases on a molecular level. As understanding of these processes continues to evolve, it segues into taking what has been understood in the laboratory setting and applying this to a clinical environment. The knowledge gained in the clinical setting can now be progressed to a community health model to provide patients with evidence-based preventions and treatments.

In the foot and ankle, translational research had its inception in cadaveric specimens. This initially provided an appreciation of anatomic variations within the foot and ankle, along with potential clinical implications of surgical procedures. With evolving research techniques, a transition from static to relatively dynamic cadaver models was able to provide further evidence towards the functional biomechanics and kinematics associated with multiple bones, ligaments, muscles, tendons, and joints of the foot and ankle. An example of this early work consisted of identifying the axes of rotation of the subtalar and midtarsal joints. The hindfoot was fixed, while the midfoot motion was traced with rods and pointers "bolted" to bones.[6] This was not without limitation, however, and it became clear that there was likely relatively limited clinical application of these findings. This stimulated translational research to begin developing a better comprehension of the complex and foundational interplay between biology and mechanics in the foot and ankle.[7] Multi-segmental models began to provide new insights into how the small and often assumed minor articulations in the foot move and function.[8] Additionally, statistical shape modeling has begun to be utilized as a computational tool to assess the three-dimensional anatomical shape and deformity of bones of the foot and ankle.[9]

Translational research of the foot and ankle has also progressed in the area of basic science with genome sequencing and the development of advanced interventional technologies. Next-generation sequencing was utilized for species-specific diagnosis of infected diabetic foot ulcerations and demonstrated high concordance rates between conventional culture and next-generation sequencing, with fair concordance observed between newly synthesized antibodies immunoassay versus culture and next-generation sequences.[10] Our understanding of human disease on a molecular level also enhanced the understanding of diabetic bone healing with Naltrexone treatment in a type 1 diabetic rat fracture model.[11] The fractured bone healing was accelerated and Naltrexone protected against some elements of compromised bone composition.

Finite element analysis is a computational model used to quantify parameters in geometrically complex structures such as the foot and ankle. This might provide evidence specific to proposed treatments of pathomechanical conditions including progressive collapsing flatfoot deformity, hallux valgus, hallux rigidus, plantar fasciitis, diabetic foot tissue loss, ankle arthritis, and lesser toe deformities.[12]

Translational research in the foot and ankle continues to provide new instruments for research that lead to discoveries extending from the laboratory to clinical application in patients. The prerequisite for the translational research model requires a focus on specific musculoskeletal diseases. Once focused findings are obtained, research skills must be developed for the bench, in the lab, and in the clinical setting. Once this is achieved, cross-disciplinary interactions between clinicians and scientists are mandatory.[13] The subsequent production of peer-reviewed publications and consensus statements are the product of translational research that impacts the community at large.

Cadaveric investigational models

One of the most challenging aspects of podiatric science is the dynamic and functional nature of the foot and ankle. This inherently makes the performance of in vivo investigations difficult if not impossible. A prime example of this challenge is represented by the "classic" 1976 article by Ramsey and Hamilton entitled "Changes in Tibiotalar Area of Contact Caused by Lateral Talar Shift."[14] The authors appropriately wanted to investigate how ankle fractures might change the anatomic alignment of the ankle joint. However, although a perfectly reasonable clinical question and hypothesis, this is not something that can be effectively measured in vivo. Perhaps interestingly in neither 1976 nor in 2024! So instead the authors had to rely on 23 amputated limbs which were dissected, disarticulated, and marked with black carbon (**Fig. 1**). This indirectly was able to provide an objective measure of tibiotalar contact with varying degrees of lateral talar displacement under the tibial plafond. Even today similar clinical questions with respect to joint space contact pressures can only be inferred indirectly based on static joint space, perhaps most accurately with weight-bearing CT scans.

Critical readers and investigators should take into consideration several important concepts when considering cadaveric methodologies. The first is whether or not the utilized cadavers are formalin-fixed embalmed or fresh frozen specimens. Formalin-fixed embalmed specimens are perhaps more readily available and less expensive, but the nature of the embalming process is certain to have an effect on soft tissue and bone biomechanical properties.[15] This is, to some degree, a confounding variable in that it is known to have some effect, but the actual effect is not completely

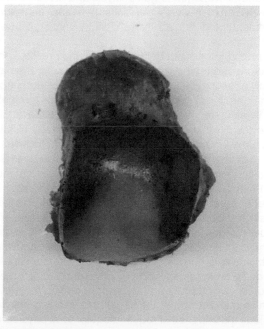

Fig. 1. Carbon marked talar dome.

understood. Fresh frozen specimens, on the other hand, might be more accurate from a tissue property standpoint, but one must ensure that proper thawing protocols were undertaken prior to experimentation.

A second consideration is loading protocols intended to mimic weight-bearing stance and other varying aspects of the gait cycle. Cadaveric methodologies likely have more clinical application if attempting to recreate closed-chain versus open-chain circumstances. Many specimens are disarticulated below the knee and therefore not completely representative of closed-chain kinetics of the lower extremity. One must consider the axial load imparted through the tibia during testing and how this load is specifically employed. Further, one must consider the effect of extrinsic tendons on the stability of the foot and ankle complex and how these might be reliably replicated. Christensen and colleagues have produced arguably the best description of this process in their cadaveric series on the biomechanics of the first ray.[16–20]

And a third consideration is whether or not the surrounding soft tissues have been dissected and stripped off of the anatomy of interest. Joints and other anatomic structures do not function in isolation. One of the marvels of the foot and ankle is the balance created between external kinematic forces and the internal support structures created by the specific anatomy of the joint surfaces, relatively static capsular and fascial structures, and relatively dynamic musculotendinous structures. The dissection process utilized to expose an anatomic area of interest for investigation might adversely affect this balance.

Cadaveric specimens perhaps allow foot and ankle scientists to most closely investigate in vivo structural anatomy and dynamic function, but this is not without inherent limitation which affects the applicability and interpretation of results.

Gait analysis and pressure measurement

A step beyond cadaveric investigations is the use of gait analysis and pressure measurement assessment. Advantages to gait analysis and pressure measurement methodologies include dynamic in-vivo data collection and analysis, objective force distribution assessment, and the ability to directly measure change following an intervention.[21]

For example, an investigator might be interested in the pressure underneath the first metatarsal head before and after a metatarsal osteotomy for the hallux valgus deformity. This is certainly a reasonable clinical question as sub-metatarsal pain and callus formation are common clinical complaints in patients with forefoot deformity. Jung and colleagues[22] investigated this question utilizing a cadaveric methodology as reviewed in the previous section. This was able to effectively simulate the effects of a metatarsal osteotomy on plantar pressures. However, Puchner and colleagues[23] added further precision to this clinical question by more directly evaluating the plantar pressures of 25 patients during gait before and after the performance of a first metatarsal osteotomy. Plantar pressures were measured in both study designs, by while the Jung and colleagues methodology was indirectly simulated in cadavers, the Puchner and colleagues methodology provided a more direct measure of outcomes by utilizing patients actually undergoing the osteotomy and actively participating in gait.

As another example, an investigator might be interested in studying the effects of an ankle brace on subjects with chronic ankle instability. Stotz and colleagues[24] investigated this clinical question, and were able to provide the direct measurement of dynamic anatomic outcomes with a gait analysis methodology.

Disadvantages and inherent limitations to gait analysis and pressure measurement methodologies include the expense of required equipment, physical space constraints to allow for effective data collection with motion capture systems, the learning curve and expertise needed to work with the software and equipment, and extrapolation and clinical application of relatively unique outcome measures[25–27] (**Fig. 2**).

Critical readers of these methodologies should familiarize themselves with the validity of specific equipment and data collection protocols, evaluate whether the study authors have sufficient expertise and experience in the field, and familiarize themselves with the clinical application of the mechanical outcome measures. For example, a common outcome measure within this methodological subset is the Newton. A "Newton (N)" is defined as the force required to accelerate one kilogram of mass at a rate of one meter per second squared, while a "Newton meter (Nm)" is a measurement of torque resulting from one Newton of force applied to a one-meter moment arm.[27] These might not be easily conceptualized nor readily applicable in terms of clinical evaluation.

With that said, however, any foot and ankle surgeon is able to develop a better understanding of these units without having to dive too deeply into the principles of physics. In fact, it is not much more complicated than the more familiar formula: Pressure = Force/Area. Put simply, higher forces and smaller areas lead to increased pressure. The Newton unit of force is somewhat more complex in that it involves the extra dimensions of speed and distance, but the general concept is the same. Higher

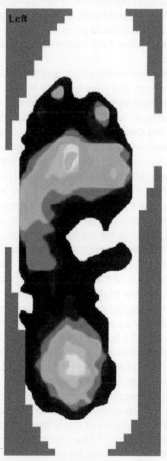

Fig. 2. Plantar pressure analysis data collection.

weights, faster speeds, and greater distances of structure contraction/extension all lead to higher force when considering the Newton. The inherent value of the unit is that it is a more dynamic and responsive measure of force, and of course the foot and ankle is a very dynamic functional anatomic area with varying forces exerted through numerous anatomic structures and in a variety of clinical situations.

Dermatology

There is a plethora of dermatological research published on a weekly basis. Ranging from therapeutic studies to quality-of-life reviews, these articles mostly cover inflammatory skin conditions, infections, and skin cancers. As an example, clinical trials for biologic agents that manage psoriasis focus on the reduction of body surface area involvement and the investigator's scoring of its success in reducing visible disease. Unfortunately, most of these studies do not isolate the feet; specifically toenails or plantar skin. The foot might be grouped in with the lower extremity or with the hands (ie, palmar/plantar). This makes the extrapolation of the data extremely difficult. Also, many subjects who are enrolled in these studies have a majority of the body affected, but might not have hand or foot involvement. Hand/foot involvement in inflammatory skin conditions is often a separate presentation of the disease state; therefore, potentially not as important to focus on compared to the more common form. Nail disease may not focus on the toenails in these studies since the fingernails are more commonly involved. However, in the author's clinical practice, having data that supports the use of these medications for the plantar foot disease and toenail involvement would be incredibly useful and impactful.

Another barrier in dermatological research is the difficulty in performing nail clinical trials. Toenails grow 1-2 mm/month and may take 12-18 months to grow from cuticle to distal tip. This makes clinical trials to study new antifungal agents lengthy, costly, and challenging. Also, there are no head-to-head studies that compare one topical antifungal agent to another and no studies demonstrating the utilization of both an oral and topical antifungal agent for onychomycosis treatment. Beyond that, one cannot compare the FDA-approved topical antifungal agents in a systematic fashion as they all define terms differently and were performed differently from a protocol perspective. The only consistent factor across the antifungal trials is mycological cure, which is defined as negative KOH and fungal culture. This is an FDA protocol mandate and does not translate to what most clinicians do in practice, which is ordering PAS stain or PCR testing to determine fungal presence. In addition, there is no standard way of calculating or assessing the recurrence of fungal disease following antifungal therapy so anecdotal numbers of recurrence are wide-ranging. Performing a study to assess recurrence would be costly and very lengthy since fungal infections of the nail tend to be insidious in nature.

When reviewing phase III clinical trials for tinea pedis, critical readers should note that they are approved for interdigital tinea which some consider the most common form of tinea pedis. Moccasin tinea pedis is very relevant in clinical practice, but there are no guidelines in place to treat it topically or systemically. No consensus has ever been reached to define what moccasin tinea pedis is and the length of time needed to treat it This creates an issue with clinical trial protocols and approval statements in the package inserts. If there is no definition of moccasin tinea pedis, then it can't be fully studied or given approval for therapy by the FDA. In a article by one of the authors (TCV), a post hoc analysis was completed for the use of naftifine gel 2% for the treatment of moccasin tinea pedis in a phase III study that encompassed tinea pedis in the interdigital space and the plantar foot.[28] The medication was FDA approved for interdigital tinea but also showed effectiveness for moccasin in this post hoc analysis. The article states, "Moccasin tinea pedis is a more severe and chronic form of the infection...with the presence of scale and hyperkeratosis."[28] The addition of hyperkeratotic lesions, often seen with plantar skin conditions, makes a superficial dermatophyte infection more of a challenge to manage. Podiatric physicians feel comfortable with the thickened stratum corneum; however, most practitioners do not and are unsure of what is necessary to treat these lower extremity conditions.

Dermatologic research that solely focuses on plantar foot, toenails, or lower extremity in general is uncommon. This requires the practitioner to extrapolate data to determine therapeutic options and read articles carefully to find if the foot was effectively considered in the protocol.

Databases

The use of large databases of deidentified patient information has become increasingly prevalent in the podiatric literature in recent years. There are several advantages to this: relatively standardized clinical definitions and data collection, large sample sizes, multicenter and multiregional data availability, ease of access, data extraction and analysis, and so forth. One representative example of this is the National Surgical Quality Improvement Program (NSQIP) database founded by the American College of Surgeons (ACS).[29–32]

With that said, this type of methodology also presents with a unique set of inherent limitations. Primary among these is that the investigators effectively "buy in" to the database and have little to no control with respect to the specific intervention and treatment of individual patients, definitions of outcome measures, included outcome measures, accuracy of data extraction, and so forth. Additionally, database studies are inherently retrospective and therefore are at risk for confounding selection bias.

This "buy in" is an interesting concept and one in which our profession should pay particular attention. Generally speaking, hospital systems pay a subscription annual fee to participate in a given database. They are effectively agreeing to include their patients within the database, and have their employees input the data with respect to individual patients. This is typically coordinated and facilitated through electronic medical record systems. With this commitment, however, the hospital system and its employees are now granted access to the entirety of the database.

So this might be advantageous to those foot and ankle surgeons who practice in large academic hospital systems, but likely is not for those who are in private practice and perform a large percentage of their surgical volume in private surgical centers.

It is also an area where our professional can likely organize and mobilize moving forward. Foot and ankle surgery-specific databases might be developed allowing for reasonable "buy in" for those in all practice situations. Foot and ankle surgery ranges from small private practices to large practice conglomerations to academic health care centers. The inclusion of patients and data from all of these differing sites is important for our profession to move itself forward in contemporary medical science. Our national organizations should have a role to help organize this and increase access for all podiatric surgeons.

DISCLOSURE

The authors have nothing to disclose related to this material.

REFERENCES

1. Olshansky SJ, Goldman DP, Zheng Y, et al. Aging in America in the twenty-first century: demographic forecasts from the MacArthur foundation research network on an aging society. Milbank Q 2009;87(4):842–62.

2. Yelin E, Weinstein S, King T. The burden of musculoskeletal diseases in the United States. Semin Arthritis Rheum 2016;46(3):259–60.
3. National Institutes of Health. Definitions under Subsection 1 (Research Objectives), Section I (Funding Opportunity Description), Part II (Full Text of Announcement), of RFA-RM-07-007: Institutional Clinical and Translational Science Award (U54). Available at: http://grants.nih.gov/grants/guide/rfa-files/RFA-RM-07-007.html. Accessed June 15, 2023.
4. Rubio DM, Schoenbaum EE, Lee LS, et al. Defining translational research: implications for training. Acad Med 2010;85(3):470–5.
5. Qin L, Chen CH, Genant HK, et al. The impact of translational orthopaedic research: journal of orthopaedic translation indexed in science citation index expanded. J Orthop Translat 2018;3(12):A1–2.
6. Manter JT. Movements of the subtalar and transverse tarsal joints. Anat Rec 1941;80:397–410.
7. Anderson DD. Upping our research game. Foot Ankle Clin N Am 2023;1:xvii–xviii.
8. Nester CJ. Lessons from dynamic cadaver and invasive bone pin studies: do we know how the foot really moves during gait? J Foot Ankle Res 2009;27(2):18.
9. Lenz AL, Lisonbee RJ. Biomechanical insights afforded by shape modeling in the foot and ankle. Foot Ankle Clin 2023;28(1):63–76.
10. Choi Y, Oda E, Waldman O, et al. Next-generation sequencing for pathogen identification in infected foot ulcers. Foot Ankle Orthop 2021;6(3). 24730114211026933.
11. Titunick MB, Lewis GS, Cain JD, et al. Blockade of the OGF-OGFr pathway in diabetic bone. Connect Tissue Res 2019;60(6):521–9.
12. Malakoutikhah H, Latt LD. Disease-specific finite element analysis of the foot and ankle. Foot Ankle Clin 2023;28(1):155–72.
13. Jacobs JJ. Translational research: whither the ORS? J Orthop Res 2008;26(5):737–40.
14. Ramsey PL, Hamilton W. Changes in tibiotalar area of contact caused by lateral talar shift. J Bone Joint Surg Am 1976;58(3):356–7.
15. Comert A, Kokat AM, Akkocaoglu M, et al. Fresh-frozen vs. embalmed bone: is it possible to use formalin-fixed human bone for biomechanical experiments on implants? Clin Oral Implants Res 2009;20(5):521–5.
16. Johnson CH, Christensen JC. Biomechanics of the first ray. Part I. The effects of peroneus longus function: a three-dimensional kinematic study on a cadaver model. J Foot Ankle Surg 1999;38(5):313–21.
17. Rush SM, Christensen JC, Johnson CH. Biomechanics of the first ray. Part II: metatarsus primus varus as a cause of hypermobility. A three-dimensional kinematic analysis in a cadaver model. J Foot Ankle Surg 2000;39(2):68–77.
18. Bierman RA, Christensen JC, Johnson CH. Biomechanics of the first ray. Part III. Consequences of Lapidus arthrodesis on peroneus longus function: a three-dimensional kinematic analysis in a cadaver model. J Foot Ankle Surg 2011;40(3):125–31.
19. Roling BA, Christensen JC, Johnson CH. Biomechanics of the first ray. Part IV: the effect of selected medial column arthrodesis. A three-dimensional kinematic analysis in a cadaver model. J Foot Ankle Surg 2002;41(5):278–85.
20. Johnson CH, Christensen JC. Biomechanics of the first ray part V: the effect of equinus deformity. A 3-dimensional kinematic study on a cadaver model. J Foot Ankle Surg 2005;44(2):114–20.
21. Hulleck AA, Mohan CM, Abdallah N, et al. Present and future of gait assessment in clinical practice: towards the application of novel trends and technologies. Front Med Technol 2022;16(4):901331.

22. Jung HG, Zaret DI, Parks BG, et al. Effect of first metatarsal shortening and dorsiflexion osteotomies on forefoot plantar pressure in a cadaver model. Foot Ankle Int 2005;26(9):748–53.
23. Puchner SE, Trnka HJ, Willegger M, et al. Comparison of plantar pressure distribution and functional outcome after Scarf and Austin osteotomy. Orthop Surg 2018;10(3):255–63.
24. Storz A, John C, Gmachowski RAL, et al. Effects of elastic ankle support on running ankle kinematics in individuals with chronic ankle instability and healthy controls. Gait Posture 2021;87:149–55.
25. Pirozzi K, McGuire J, Meyr AJ. A comparison of two total contact cast constructs with variable body mass. J Wound Care 2014;23(Suppl 7):S4–14.
26. Pirozzi K, McGuire J, Meyr AJ. Effect of variable body mass on plantar foot pressure and off-loading device efficacy. J Foot Ankle Surg 2014;53(5):588–97.
27. Mateen S, Sansosti LE, Meyr AJ. A critical biomechanical evaluation of foot and ankle soft tissue repair. Clin Podiatr Med Surg 2022;39(3):521–33.
28. Stein Gold LF, Vlahovic T, Verma A, et al. Natifine hydrochloride gel 2%: an effective topical treatment for moccasin-type tinea pedis. J Drugs Dermatol 2015;14(10):1138–44.
29. Meyr AJ, Sansosti LE. An evaluation of basic demographic characteristics in foot and ankle surgery from the American college of surgeons national surgical quality improvement program. J Foot Ankle Surg 2022;61(5):996–1000.
30. Meyr AJ, Dougherty M, Kwaadu KY. An evaluation of patient characteristics associated with medical disposition in the surgical treatment of ankle fractures. J Foot Ankle Surg 2022;61(1):72–8.
31. Meyr AJ, Skolnik J, Mateen S, et al. A comparison of adverse short-term outcomes following forefoot amputation performed on an inpatient versus outpatient basis. J Foot Ankle Surg 2022;61(1):67–71.
32. Meyr AJ, Mateen S, Skolnik J, et al. Evaluation of the relationship between aspects of medical complexity and work relative value units (wRVUs) for foot and ankle surgical procedures. J Foot Ankle Surg 2021;60(3):448–54.

Working with Industry

Adam S. Landsman, DPM, PhD*

KEYWORDS

- Consulting • Investigator sponsored studies • Industry • Biomedical engineering

KEY POINTS

- Benefits and drawbacks of Industry participation in medical science.
- Conflict of Interest statements are important.
- The role of physicians in Industry sponsored research.
- Entering the world of biomedical consulting and research as a young physician/scientist.

INTRODUCTION

In 1992, I completed a 9-year dual-degree program where I received both my DPM degree and a PhD in Bioengineering. Upon my graduation, it was apparent that "Industry" had an interest in me. Sponsored research and consulting opportunities where readily available, and I had to learn very quickly to sort the scientific from the sham, and the clinically worthwhile from the worthless. Throughout my professional life, I have worked to some degree in Industry, in a variety of scenarios. In this article, I will share my personal experiences to try and illustrate both the benefits and pitfalls of working with Industry in a variety of scenarios.

There are a variety of ways in which a physician might work with Industry. Some of these options can be integrated into a clinical practice while others cannot. It is important to remember that Industry usually wants to work with doctors that have clinical experience and/or an educational background that can be utilized by the company. Opportunities can exist in product development, clinical research and product testing, promotional and sales activities, and regulatory work. Frequently, doctors with business training and experience may also take a lead role in business development.

For those of us who want to go beyond the direct patient care experience, working with Industry can be highly rewarding and fascinating addition to your career. In this article, we will look at how to approach various opportunities with Industry.

Clinical Trials

Clinical research funding can be difficult to secure. Federal funding can be particularly difficult as it is highly competitive and has become politicized over the years. Popular, more established scientists are likely to have an edge over young investigators, which

Division of Podiatric Surgery, Department of Orthopedic Surgery and FARIL, Massachusetts General Hospital, Harvard Medical School, Boston, MA, USA
* Massachusetts General Hospital, Yawkey 3F, 55 Fruit Street, Boston, MA 02114.
E-mail address: alandsman@mgh.harvard.edu

Clin Podiatr Med Surg 41 (2024) 343–349
https://doi.org/10.1016/j.cpm.2023.07.008
0891-8422/24/© 2023 Elsevier Inc. All rights reserved.

podiatric.theclinics.com

is why young investigator award programs exist. Even when study review panels are blinded, it might be obvious who the investigators are based on the contents of the proposal. Although I have been fortunate to have federal funding in the past, the hours required, and the number of applications that had to be submitted to achieve funding can be overwhelming. Nonetheless, there are many investigators who have no choice. Typically projects that involve the most basic science, are very early stage, or have no obvious commercial potential fall into this pool. But research involving commercial products or services may be funded in whole or in part by Industry.

Clinical trials are often privately funded by Industry or by a physician that is interfacing with Industry. Most Industry-sponsored clinical trials are managed through an organization referred to as a CRO (Clinical Research Organization) in order to satisfy approval requirements by the FDA (Food and Drug Administration). These CRO's are usually large international companies that are required to operate independently from the study sponsor. This autonomy prevents the industry sponsor from tampering with data. Physicians who would like to participate in these types of clinical trials can register with CROs online. You can discuss your specialty and the types of patients that your practice attracts (ie, diabetics, reconstruction candidates, sports injuries, and so forth) and the CRO will reach out to you when they have a study available with the type of patients that you can provide. CROs are always looking for ethical investigator clinicians. These studies are divided into phases, depending on whether they have been tried in patients previously or not.

Clinical trials of this type can be fairly time-consuming but the participating clinicians are usually very well compensated, and there are no billing or insurance hassles. These studies normally provide a stipend for the clinical investigators, and often include funding for the patients in addition to providing the patient with study drugs or devices, x-rays, lab tests, and so forth.

Industry-sponsored studies are sometimes both designed and written by the physician and are called "Investigator Initiated." Investigator-initiated studies begin with the physician reaching out to a company that produces something they are interested in studying. For example, a physician may want to determine if a dietary supplement can reduce the risk of ulcerations in poorly controlled diabetics. The physician could approach the manufacturer(s) of the dietary supplement with a proposal that describes what the research project would look like, and what funding is needed, if any. The company might be very interested if it looks like their product could be helpful in serving a population that they have not targeted in the past. In some cases, they may even retain the physician to work with members of their team to put together the study. This approach can be very exciting and satisfying for both the doctor and the company, if they discover a new way to treat an ailment, and also sell more products.

Once the research is completed, it normally is written about in a scientific journal, and goes through a peer-review process prior to publication. The investigators who performed the study are usually the ones who do this type of write-up. However, some great investigators are not great writers or simply do not have the time, and this is where the medical writer, sometimes called "ghost writer" comes in. Industry employs writers who can present complex scientific data in a concise and understandable manner. It is in their best interest to present the data in a way that demonstrates the outcomes that they invested in producing. Papers that result from sponsored research should include a disclaimer that acknowledges their input.

Consulting

When it comes to working with Industry, keep in mind that you have expertise that is highly desirable, and you have spent many long years to gather that information.

Consultants impart their knowledge and expertise for a fee, to someone who needs it. However, it is not always obvious how to get a company to recognize the value that you bring. It is up to you to demonstrate this to them, but how? You can share your expertise through obvious channels, such as lecturing or writing on your strongest topics. Frequently, these activities will lead to a company finding you.

You can also engage with a company by asking questions. In his book, *What Clients Love; A Field Guide to Growing Your Business*, by Harry Beckwith,[1] he advises that companies are attracted to consultants who make their interests in a company or product known. They speak with Medical Directors and other Consultants, about their interests. They familiarize themselves with the product line and the company. They share willingly and freely in the beginning so that the company can appreciate the value of their wisdom and enthusiasm.

A good consultant should have a clear picture of what they can bring to the company – clinical insights, useful design modifications, ideas to expand a company's market share, or even ways to reduce costs of a product. Good consultants also should be very involved in their field of interest. They attend conferences. They walk through all the booths where the vendors are and ask lots of questions.

Throughout my career, I will look at a category of products, and try to define what differentiates them from one another within that category. For example, if you are considering biologic materials for wound care, you should understand what your options are, and try to define broad categories to group these products. Specifically, one might consider hypothesized mechanisms of action, composition, FDA classification, costs, indications, and even availability in the region. Once you understand the field and who the players are, you can help your clients to strategize and differentiate their products from the others. You can potentially repurpose their product to broaden the appeal and increase market shares. You may even be able to help them modify their product for other purposes, and this is where Product Development comes into focus.

Product Development

Once you have become an expert in your field, you will inevitably think of a way to do things better, faster, and with less complications and expenses. I find new product development (or sometimes new product acquisition) to be the most exciting and rewarding type of Industry interaction.

The FDA (Food and Drug Administration) utilizes a five step process for medical device development.[2] These steps are clearly outlined on their web page and involve the following sections.

1. Device Discovery and Concept
2. Preclinical Research and Prototyping
3. Initiation of Approval Pathway
4. Device review by the FDA
5. Post-Market Device Safety Monitoring by the FDA

Since the goal of Medical Product Development will inevitably involve the FDA, it is always advisable to implement your ideas these guidelines in mind.

While working with a company that processed implantable collagen, I was asked to use their existing material for reconstructing tendons. The product I began with was already in use by plastic surgeons for breast augmentation. The idea was to cut the existing material differently to alter the thickness and shape in order to make it more flexible and also easier to incorporate into the injured tissue. The modified product was perfectly suited for tendon repair, and the company ended up selling more collagen for soft tissue reconstruction then for breast augmentation.

Sometimes product development involves the modification of an existing product, and at other times, starting with a completely clean slate to create something new and different. In other cases, product development involves the purchase of another company or product line that can be modified to meet the needs of your company.

Product development also has the added benefit of potentially bringing you royalties, stock options, equity, and other methods of delayed payment. Whenever a clinician/consultant has a financial stake in a particular product, it is essential that this be explicitly disclosed to any patient that you might treat using that product. Also, there have been times when the consultant already holds intellectual property or a pending patent, and in this case, separate negotiations are needed to protect the rights of all parties – Industry, who will likely be funding the product or idea, and the Inventor.

Medical Directorship

Medical directors have the responsibility of making sure that products are used properly, and in a safe and efficacious manner. This role usually involves the development or refinement of treatment protocols, while remaining within the boundaries set by regulatory agencies and in some cases the FDA. Frequently, the Medical Director is in charge of fielding questions from physicians regarding their company's products and services. The Medical Director typically works very closely with the sales and marketing team, to help identify the market and craft the sales message. Often times, it is the Medical Director who will determine that focused research is needed, and may even write or oversee the development and implementation of clinical trials.

Depending on the size of the company and the responsibilities of the director, this often something that can be done on a part-time basis, in conjunction with clinical practice. In this way, the Medical Director can stay current with the state of knowledge in their field. Some companies may employ more than one Director in order to focus their efforts are various markets.

Bedenkov, and colleagues[3] published an interesting summary of the responsibilities and duties of a Medical Director in Industry. They should bring a broad skill set to the enterprise, including creativity, patient centricity, prioritization, and leadership. Medical Directors, have a broad understanding of the science and existing technology in their arena, and must be capable of building a team and possibly drawing from outside experts to build to support their company's goals.

Medical Directors have widely ranging roles from company to company. They are part of the executive team but their duties can range from product creation to dealing with regulatory issues, to responding to technical inquiries from physician customers. In an excellent article in the magazine, Wired, an article by Wolf[4] described Steve Jobs' creative role at Apple. One thing that is obvious, is that Jobs had an amazing ability to understand what attracted customers, and where the market was going. Certainly the term, visionary applies here. Good Medical Directors fall in to this role of liaison between the Corporate Board, Scientists, Sales teams, and Physicians, and can help to direct the company to develop the right technologies and get them to the desired customers.

Marketing and the Continuing Medical Education Lectures

Many doctors and other medical personnel become involved in Industry through lecturing and market promotion. Most of us have attended a dinner lecture or sponsored conference presentation at some time where an expert in the field will discuss their experiences with a product or service. These lecturers are very knowledgeable in their field, and are there to educate us in an area of interest that is usually somehow connected to an Industry leader. In some cases, it is forbidden to present information that specifically supports a product or service. The CME (Continuing Medical Education) lecture should be free of any commercial or promotional activities, and presenters are supposed to state unambiguously if they have any affiliation or conflicts of interest with the presentation sponsor(s). The FDA has strict rules regarding what can and cannot be said in a CME program[5] and frequently these presentations are discretely monitored. Many companies will develop highly scripted lectures that make sure that the presentations are presented in accordance with official guidelines, and may even require the presentation to be reviewed by their legal team before being given.

Promotional lectures are usually designed to teach the attendees about a condition or disease state, and present a product that the lecturer is familiar with that helps to manage this condition or disease state. In some cases, these lectures may involve several products or classes of products, and then may compare and contrast them based on the lecturer's experiences as well as data from the clinical literature. In my experience, these lectures are usually quite informative and help me to understand as both a clinician and as a consultant exactly what the mission is of a particular industry. They are laying out what they feel are the needs of the health care providers, and showing us exactly what their treatment strategy is.

Consider the Lapidus bunionectomy. This is a procedure that has gone through a renaissance over the last 10 years, driven by doctors and consultants who felt that frontal plane rotation and medial column instability surrounding the first metatarsal was not being well managed by existing surgical approaches. This was their message, and the solution conveniently came from Industry that provided new instrumentation and new internal fixation devices to solve the problem. The message was delivered through well-constructed scientific studies,[6-8] which led to multiple lectures and presentations at national venues and local meetings, as well as training courses, industry-sponsored certification, and even direct-to-consumer advertisements. The Lapidus bunionectomy is a good procedure that has helped many patients, and has become a favorite among foot surgeons of all types. To me, the amazing part is that this procedure was first described by Dr. Lapidus in 1934, but did not rise to its current level of popularity until 75 years later! This is also a great example of how Industry, Consultants, Clinicians, and Marketers can work together to create a new niche in this profession, while reshaping the way we think about a common ailment and at the same time, providing a solution that has obviously been successful.

Often times, promotional lectures may be extended into hands-on training through cadaver labs, working with models, and even "certification" in a technique that might be particularly labor intensive or technique dependent. These types of hands-on training sessions are frequently created and taught by clinicians who are hired by Industry. In some cases, the inventors or developers of the new technology may also be the instructor. Experts with knowledge of the nuances of utilization lead these courses, whether it is the sequence used to drill a bone, or the best way to secure a graft. By becoming proficient with a particular device, you may be able to work with Industry to become a KOL – a Key Opinion Leader.

Key Opinion Leaders's and Advisory Boards

Key Opinion Leaders are clinicians with a strong reputation in their area of interest as a thought leader. The role of KOLs is to advise Industry on the best places to use their products, and to advise them on the distinctions between the company's products and their competitors. KOLs may help to promote a company's product in many ways including product development and refinement, creation of clinical trials, creating "slide decks," and group authorship of scientific findings. KOLs are there to advise a company on how best to address the KOL's colleagues, in order to improve and promote their products.

Sales force training is another area where Industry may rely upon your clinical expertise. In the past, I have been called upon to give presentations to various sales forces and executives in Industry, to enlighten them on how their products and their competitor's products are accepted in the field. Competing studies must be analyzed and presented so that all can understand the advantages and disadvantages that they should expect to encounter. Sometimes this may even lead to presentations to regulatory agencies, where they are trying to ascertain similarities and differences between products that are new and products that are already approved (ie, predicate devices). This type of information is also frequently used by industry to convince insurance carriers to approve their products for coverage. Most of the time, Industry employs people who are experts in negotiating these Federal guidelines. In some cases, clinicians may be hired to consult with attorneys and regulatory experts.

The Down Side of Industry Collaboration

I have always found working with Industry to be one of the most enjoyable aspects of my professional career. It has afforded me the opportunity to dive in deeply in my areas of interest, to write and implement clinical trials, and author peer-reviewed articles. Industry has also opened the door to me to develop and produce products and services that have been widely used by many of my colleagues. It is incredibly exciting to sit in a room of engineers and scientists, and develop a new product or tool from scratch, and see it actually grow through the approval process to end up on an actual patient. There is a tremendous amount of pride that comes with seeing someone whose health has been improved by an idea that I had that actually became a product.

However, in the world of Industry consulting, you have chosen to align yourself with a business interest, and this comes at a cost. There is a perception that you are a "hired gun" which is someone that will do or say anything as long as the money keeps coming in. Those of us that work in Industry on a regular basis have to be prepared for this type of criticism. If you let your name and your expertise be attached to a product or service, it should be done with a clear head, because you truly believe in the data and the product itself that you are supporting. At the end of the day, the best KOLs are the ones who present accurate and meaningful data in an honest way. Clinicians want to provide the best for their patients, and it is prudent for the KOL/Researcher/Industry Representative to be forthright in the benefits and shortcomings of their products.

Unfortunately, many KOLs become synonymous with their Industry partners, and are no longer viewed as reliable sources. This is a double-edged opportunity because on one side, it is great to be considered a true expert in your field, but not at the cost of being a one-sided company puppet. For this reason, transparent disclosures and conflicts of interest are critical for the clinician who frequently works for industry. You have to remember to preserve your independence of thought while working for Industry, or run the risk of becoming another sales person. It is important to discuss your Industry sponsor as well as their competitors and their points of view, ultimately to the benefit of our patients searching for a cure.

SUMMARY

Interactions with the biomedical Industry can take on many forms, ranging from Key Opinion Leader to Clinical Researcher to Medical Director. Each of these positions requires a different skill set and level of clinical experiences. There are numerous opportunities to interact with industry in order to reach your goals, whether they are financial, intellectual, or improving care for your patients. As with any professional opportunity, you should strive for improvements in quality, while maintaining transparency in both your thought process and financial arrangements in order to avoid any potential conflicts of interest. Interactions with Industry can help to broaden your own understanding of various clinical problems, and may lead you to develop or introduce new clinical treatment options for patients around the world.

CLINICS CARE POINTS

- The opportunities to work with Industry are widely varied and can range from consulting to research to product development to sales and directorship.

- Collaboration with Industry should be based on a mutual goal of bringing the best, most scientifically valid ideas to your profession, to give the best possible care to your patients.

- Industry can offer many ways for a physician to expand their activities outside of the clinic to help the entire profession by advancing the science of your specialty.

- There are many ways for physicians tied to Industry to earn extra income, and it is important to remain transparent about your affiliations to maintain your integrity as a physician and scientist.

DISCLOSURE

The author has no conflicts of interest to disclose related to this article. The author has consulted in the past for Misonix, Soluble Systems, Bioventus, Blossom Innovations, Urgo Medical, Ossio, Kent Camera, Defender Operations, Enzysurge, Crossroads Extremity Systems, Medline Industries, Oculus Innovative Sciences, NuvoLase, NeuroTherm, AFCell, Nomir Medical, TEI Biosciences, The Good Feet Store, Wright Medical, Novartis, LifeNet Health, KMI, Smith + Nephew, and Pfizer.

REFERENCES

1. Beckwith H. What Clients Love: A field guide to growing your business. Business Plus; 2010. ASIN: 0446556025; ISBN-10: 9780446556026.
2. https://www.fda.gov/patients/learn-about-drug-and-device-approvals/device-development-process
3. Bedenkov A, Rajadhyaksha V, Moreno C, et al. The 7+ habits of highly effective medical directors. Pharm Med 2021;35:267–79.
4. Wood, G; Steve Jobs: The Next Insanely Great Thing, Available at:https://www.wired.com/1996/02/jobs-2/.
5. https://www.fda.gov/regulatory-information/search-fda-guidance-documents/industry-supported-scientific-and-educational-activities
6. Dayton P, Hatch DJ, Santrock RD, et al. Biomechanical characteristics of biplane multiplanar tension-side fixation for Lapidus fusion. J Foot Ankle Surg 2018;57(4):766–70.
7. Smith WB, Dayton P, Santrock RD, et al. Understanding frontal plane correction in hallux valgus repair. Clin Podiatr Med Surg 2018;35(1):27–36.
8. Feilmeier M, Dayton P, Kauwe M, et al. Comparison of transverse and coronal plane stability at the first tarsal-metatarsal joint with multiple screw orientations. Foot Ankle Spec 2017;10(2):104–8.

Effective Manuscript Preparation and Submission

Donald Scot Malay, DPM, MSCE

KEYWORDS

- Electornic search terms • Journal's guidefor authors • Publication
- Report of scientific research

KEY POINTS

- Preparation of an ideal manuscript.
- One key to getting the journal editors to accept a report is that the manuscript is properly organized and in compliance with the journal's Guide for Authors.
- If the subject matter is interesting and scientifically rigorous, then a well-written manuscript that complies with the journal's requirements will likely cruise through the peer review process and get accepted for publication.

TITLE PAGE

The title page should include the title of the report, a list of the authors and their credentials written precisely how each author wants to be represented, and the authors' contact and conflict of interest (disclosures) information. The corresponding author should be clearly identified, and it is that individual's responsibility to keep the coauthors informed of peer reviewers' and editors' critical appraisals and recommendations (reject, revise, accept). The title, as provided in the title page, will be used in any publication related to the article, as will the order of the authors submitted. The title should unambiguously describe the subject of the report and the method of scientific inquiry used to procure the results.

LEVEL OF CLINICAL EVIDENCE

Immediately following the Abstract, the level of clinical evidence (LOCE) should be stated in accordance with the levels depicted in **Table 1**. For reports of original research, levels 1 to 3 are appropriate, if the scientific rigor of the investigation adequately limits biases that could threaten the validity of the authors' conclusions.

Penn Presbyterian Medical Center, 3801 Filbert Streeet, Medical Office Building, Suite 111, Philadelpha, PA 19004, USA
E-mail address: malaydsm@gmail.com

Clin Podiatr Med Surg 41 (2024) 351–358
https://doi.org/10.1016/j.cpm.2023.08.004
0891-8422/24/© 2023 Elsevier Inc. All rights reserved.

podiatric.theclinics.com

Table 1		
Levels of clinical evidence[a]		
Level	Type of Report	Description
1	Randomized controlled trial (RCT)	Interventional clinical experiment, hypothesis testing
2	Cohort study (prospective or retrospective)	Observational, hypothesis generating
3	Case-control study	
4	Case series or report	
5	Expert opinion, animal, or benchtop study	

[a] This table is arranged from top to bottom, beginning with the research design most likely to produce valid conclusions, namely the randomized controlled trial, to the research designs least likely to produce valid conclusions regarding human clinical outcomes, namely expert opinion, and animal or benchtop investigations.

KEY WORDS

Authors should provide three to five key words or phrases for indexing purposes, keeping in mind that electronic searches of the biomedical literature depend to a large degree on key words (refer to PubMed's Medical Subject Heading webpage for help selecting key words [http://www.ncbi.nlm.nih.gov, accessed 08/18/2023]). Avoid abbreviations in the key words unless a proprietary name uses an abbreviation, and, in general, proper names are not used as key words. As previously noted, do not repeat words or terms in the list of key words that are already stated in the title, because this reduces the opportunity to use different words that could be included in electronic searches, thus diminishing the likelihood of an electronic link (hit) to your published report.

DISCLOSURES

Immediately following designation of the LOCE, the author should disclose any financial support for the investigation and then disclose potential conflicts of interest. If there was no financial support, and if there were no conflicts of interest, then the author should write: "Financial Disclosure: None reported. Conflict of Interest: None reported."

TEXT OF THE REPORT

The text of an original research report generally consists of the following four sections: Introduction, Patients/Materials and Methods, Results, and Discussion.

Introduction

This section provides a concise overview of the state of knowledge regarding the specific problem being studied. It starts with a statement of the problem and its clinical/social importance, followed by an explanation of recent (past 5–10 years) and important (classic) reports related to the topic, supported by reference citations. The importance of the topic is best conveyed by means of statistics that indicate the prevalence and/or economic impact of the condition. After describing what is known and what remains unknown regarding the focus of the study, the author should state the specific research question and any hypothesis tested in the current investigation. The last sentence of the Introduction should state the primary aim and study design (see **Table 1**).

Patients/Materials and Methods

If the study is a clinical investigation involving living human participants (patients, subjects), then the heading for this section should be "Patients and Methods." If the investigation involves animals, cadavers, or in vitro models of any sort, including computer models, then this section should be termed "Materials and Methods." In essence, this section should describe how the authors used the building blocks of good clinical evidence in the investigation (**Box 1**).[1] More detailed discussions of these important elements of a biomedical investigation can be found at a number of evidence-based medicine Web sites, including the Centre for Health Evidence (http://www.cche.net/, accessed 08/18/2023) and the Oxford Centre for Evidence-based Medicine (http://www.cebm.net/, accessed 08/18/2023).

For reports of research involving human subjects, authors should indicate whether the investigation was conducted with institutional review board (IRB, sometimes termed the ethics committee) approval and the participants/patients volunteered to be in the study. IRB approval informs the journal editors that human research subjects were handled in a morally right and fair fashion. The name of the review board and the study approval number should be denoted. Participants in the investigation should be referred to as "participants" if the diagnostic test or intervention was experimental and not yet approved for use by the US Food and Drug Administration (FDA) and as patients for all other tests or interventions that are already known to be therapeutic, safe, and efficacious. If the study involved investigation of a new drug or device, then the FDA Investigational New Drug number should be provided (https://www.fda.gov/drugs/types-applications/investigational-new-drug-ind-application [accessed 08/19/2023]), and if the investigation involved a new device, then the FDA Premarket Notification or 510(k) number should be provided (https://www.fda.gov/patients/device-development-process/step-4-fda-device-review [accessed 08/19/2023]).

Ideally, the methods section should provide enough detail to allow subsequent researchers to replicate the study. When reporting randomized controlled trials (RCTs), a study flow diagram in Consolidated Standards of Reporting Trials (CONSORT) format, as well as the information required by the CONSORT checklist, should be provided (http://www.consort-statement.org and https://www.equator-network.org/[accessed 08/18/2023]). For observational studies, authors are encouraged to follow the Strengthening the Reporting of Observational Studies in Epidemiology (STROBE) guidelines (https://www.strobe-statement.org/[accessed 08/18/2023]). Ideally, authors submitting reports of clinical trials should have registered their investigation with a public domain repository, such as ClinicalTrials.gov (http://clinicaltrials.

Box 1
The building blocks of good clinical evidence

1. Explicitly defined research question, population, and end points

2. Randomized treatment allocation and intention-to-treat analysis

3. Participants and outcomes assessors blind to treatment allocation

4. Use of a valid health measurement (quality of life) instrument

5. Power and sample size determined a priori

6. Statistical analyses compatible with type and distribution of the data

7. Point estimate and 95% confidence interval reported

Adapted from Turlick MA, Kushner D, Stock D. J Am Podiatri Med Assoc 93: 392-8, 2003.

gov/[accessed 08/18/2023]), and the name of the public domain repository and the trial registration number should be denoted in the methods section of the report.

The following elements of the investigation should be concisely described in the methods section.

- Aims (primary and secondary)
- Study population
- Assessors and other members of the investigating team, population, or sample
- Interventions
- Variables (dependent variables, outcomes, and independent variables, exposures, or risk factors)
- Statistical methods used to describe the sample and to determine the meaning of the results.

Aims

The primary aim of the investigation, as well as any secondary aims, should be clearly stated. A distinction should be made between primary and secondary aims. As a rule, the sample size should be large enough to identify a statistically significant difference in outcomes related to the primary aim, if such a difference exists. Power and sample size calculations can be determined using any of several software programs, such as that found at: https://vbiostatps.app.vumc.org/ps/(accessed 08/18/2023). In describing the primary aim, it is common for authors to state that they undertook to answer the research question or test their hypothesis.

Assessors

Members of the investigational team should be described regarding their participation in the study, namely, if they served as outcome assessors, if they performed an intervention or, and if they abstracted data from medical records, in the case of a retrospective study. For studies in which subjective measurements are determined, such as measurements of radiographic angles, a method should be described for breaking ties and determining an outcome when indecision or uncertainty exists. If outcomes assessors were blind to treatment allocation, this must be stated. If outcomes assessors were participants in the intervention, such as members of the surgical team or treating clinicians, this must also be stated.

Study Population

The methods section should provide readers with an explicit description of the participant/patient population and the time from which they were selected. The period should delineate the day, month, and year that the period started; and the day, month, and year that the period ended (MM/DD/YYYY–MM/DD/YYYY). If the day that the time started is not precisely known, then it is acceptable to state just the month and year that initiated and ended the period (MM/YYYY–MM/YYYY). This is an important detail, because the duration of interest can be very different, and remains unclear, if only the year at the start and end of the time period is mentioned. For instance, 01/01/2021 to 12/31/23 (36 months) is considerably longer than 12/31/21 to 01/01/2023 (12 months and 2 days), and it would be ambiguous if the author just said the duration extended from 2021 to 2023 without at least detailing the month along with the year. It is also important to state that whether subjects from the sample were randomly allocated to a treatment arm and whether the subjects were blind to treatment allocation. For case series and cohort studies, the author should state whether the participants were enrolled consecutively, and if not consecutively, then the selection bias must be described. The inclusion and exclusion criteria must be clearly stated, and it is best to simply list these in a fashion that would allow other interested investigators to repeat your study.

Interventions

The intervention under investigation needs to be explicitly described. If participants were randomized to an active therapy that was compared with standard therapy or to placebo, then each regimen needs to be described. Authors are encouraged to avoid presenting a detailed narrative report of an operative intervention for a standard procedure that can be referenced in a textbook or published article, because the published procedure can be cited; however, variations on the procedure, as well as adjunct procedures, need to be described in detail. Novel interventions, notable variations on standard procedures, and critical decision points related to an intervention should be thoroughly described. For medications or devices used in the intervention, generic names should be used. If a proprietary term is used, the brand name should be used the first time the item is described, with the generic term denoted in parentheses. Thereafter, only the generic term should be used to avoid making the report sound like a sales pitch. The first time a brand name is stated, it must include trademarks and be followed by parentheses enclosing the manufacturer's name and headquarters address. For medications used in the study, complete dosing information (dose, method of administration, frequency, and duration of use) should be described.

Variables

As a rule, any variable that a reasonable clinician would consider important in regard the treatment of a patient, as it pertains to the investigation, should be considered in the analyses. Variables are either outcomes (dependent variables) or exposures/risk factors (independent variables). Each of these should be explicitly defined in terms of how the variable was measured, who made the measurement, and whether the assessor was blind to the intervention (for an intervention trial) or not. Authors should clearly state if variables were based on physical examination, chart review, telephone interview, questionnaire or radiographic images, or some other method.

Whenever possible, it is preferable that "hard" endpoints are used, such as analytical measurements, clinical or microbiology laboratory results, and the like. Whenever "soft" endpoints, such as quality of life (QOL) or foot related QOL, are considered, it is preferable to use health measurement instruments that have previously been shown to be reliable and to provide valid information. Keep in mind that a health measurement instrument in and of itself is not said to be valid, although the information gained from the use of the health measurement instrument may (and should) be. QOL instruments should be specific to the anatomy and function being tested. Investigator derived questionnaires should be described in terms of reliability and validity, if such testing was undertaken by the investigators, or if it has been described in a previous publication. For scales that rank categories (eg, *mild, moderate, severe*), an aggregate score should be used. For measurements of pain, the 10-cm visual analog scale is recommended.

In addition to the outcome/s of interest (dependent variable/s), typical independent variables (exposures, risk factors) include such things as age and age category, gender, activity level, body mass index (BMI) or BMI category, comorbidities, medications, duration of treatment, surgeon or clinical site, adjunct therapies, frequency and duration of follow-up, and post-intervention management procedures (immobilization, physical therapy, and so forth). Items such as those listed above should be referred to as "variables" and not as "parameters," because the term "parameter" should be reserved for statistical expressions that describe the data, such as the mean and standard deviation, or beta coefficients derived from regression analyses.

Statistical Methods

The statistical plan should be clearly described, and every investigation should include at least descriptive and inferential statistical analyses. The descriptive statistical analysis should define parameters such as the measure of central tendency (mean or median average) and measures of dispersion (standard deviation or range). The parameter, as well as the statistical test, should be selected based on the type and distribution of the data and the level of statistical significance defined. Typically, statistical significance is defined at the 5% ($P \leq .05$) level. Descriptive statistics should be used to describe the sample using means and standard deviations for normally distributed continuous data and counts and percentages for categorical data. Tests of the null hypothesis should be used to measure the association of independent variables with the outcomes of interest, using parametric tests for normally distributed data and nonparametric tests for data with skewed distributions. For cohort studies, the incidence of the outcome of interest should be calculated, and tests of the null hypothesis and univariate logistic regression used to measure associations between exposures and the outcome of interest and associations that meet statistical significance at the 10% level ($P \leq .1$), as well as those that are deemed clinically important, should be included in a multiple variable logistic regression model in an effort to adjust for interaction between independent variables and the outcome of interest. Confounding analyses should be undertaken so that beta coefficients can be compared, and changes of 10% to 15% should be considered indicative of confounding, and sensitivity analyses should be undertaken to measure the potential influence that unmeasured confounders could have on the results of cohort study analyses. If the time to an outcome of interest is measured, then Cox regression analyses, or other survival analyses, should be used to measure associations with the outcomes of interest. For meta-analyses, tests of homogeneity must be presented, and the method of and rationale for pooling data must be explained.

Results should be presented with only as much precision as is of scientific value. For example, measures of association (odds ratios, relative risks, risk differences, and so forth) should typically be reported to two significant digits. As a rule, the terms "significant" and "significantly" should be reserved for use when describing statistical differences. The statement "no significant difference was found" between two or more groups should not be made unless a power analysis was done and the value of alpha (level of significance, typically 5%) or beta (the power to detect a statistically significant difference, usually 80% or 90%) is reported.

The use of the word "significant" requires that a P-value (probability of the null) or, preferably, the 95% confidence interval about a point estimate, is reported. Ninety-five percent confidence intervals are preferred whenever the results of survivor analyses are given in the text, tables, or graphs. Except when one-sided tests are required by study methodology, such as in noninferiority trials, two-sided P-values should be reported. By convention, P-values larger than 0.01 should be reported to two decimal places, those between 0.01 and 0.001 to three decimal places, and P-values smaller than 0.001 should be reported as $P < .001$. Probabilities should never be reported as $P = .000$ or 1. Furthermore, use of the word "correlation" or the term "correlates with" requires that a correlation coefficient be calculated and reported, otherwise terms such as "association" or "associated" should be used.

The results of a sensitivity analysis, such as that described by Greenland,[2] or those described by Rosenbaum,[3,4] should be presented for retrospective studies where unmeasured independent variables may have potentially influenced the results. Additional references[5–8] that may be useful regarding the description of the methods and the presentation of a statistical plan are available to interested readers.

RESULTS

The results section should provide quantitative information about the data collected, in the form of descriptive and inferential statistics. Relevant information about the study population should be presented, including demographic information for each subgroup (control group and placebo or standard therapy groups), exclusions, and attrition. Inferential statistics should be used to compare groups using appropriate statistical tests based on the size of the study population, type of variables under study (discrete vs categorical), and the distribution of the data collected. Quantitative information should be summarized in the text, and readers should be referred to relevant tables for more detailed information. As a rule, a minimum of three results tables should be presented and designated as Table 1 and Box 1. Table 1 typically depicts the baseline demographic characteristics of the sample population, often categorizing the patients/participants by intervention or outcome and showing whether statistically significant differences existed between the groups. For RCTs, it is not necessary to depict statistically significant differences at baseline because randomization distributes the characteristics by chance. Table 2 generally depicts the results of tests of the null hypothesis for RCTs and univariate analyses for cohort studies, and Table 3 generally depicts the results of the multiple variable analyses for cohort studies, or survival analyses for time-to-event analyses. Additional tables can be helpful when the data warrant such detail.

Figures and tables used to report the results need to be complete with *enough detail to stand alone*, without the need for the reader to refer to the detailed text to fully understand the results. The sample size (with attention to the number of feet and the number of patients) should be stated in parentheses at the end of the title of the table or figure [eg, "(N = 73 feet in 61 patients)"]. Therefore, the table title, headings, and legends need to be thoughtfully phrased so that there is no ambiguity or lack of information.

For RCTs, the first figure should be the study flow chart (see CONSORT statement, above). For meta-analyses and systematic reviews, a Christmas tree diagram should be included. Consistency and clarity are required when reporting results. As a rule, report means with standard deviations (using the $\pm$ symbol) and medians with the range (either minimum and maximum or 25th and 75th percentiles) and *always* report the proportion of the whole when presenting count data [eg, "…4 (3.25%) displayed wound dehiscence…"], and report calculations to at least two decimal places. It is also crucial that authors remain clear and consistent when they report *denominators*, with a particular emphasis on clarity regarding the number of patients versus the number of feet or ankles or extremities, because these numbers vary based on unilateral versus bilateral cases.

DISCUSSION

The discussion section should describe the authors' interpretation of the results of their investigation. Authors should consider how their results fit into the general state of knowledge on the subject as well as their clinical relevance. In addition, authors should acknowledge the limitations of their investigation that may have introduced bias, and they should discuss how the results could have been affected by bias. The penultimate paragraph of the Discussion should present the limitations of the study methodology and may also include an explanation of the advantages of the investigation relative to prior studies. The final paragraph of the discussion should describe the authors' conclusions.

REFERENCES

References are cited in the body of the text by means of numeric citations listed parenthetically in the appropriate sentence, before the end of the sentence (usually just before the period ending the sentence). Reference citations are to appear in sequential numeric order, beginning with the number "1" and continuing in order the first time that a particular reference is cited, until the last citation is noted. In other words, supply references numbered in the exact order they appear in the text (not alphabetically).

ELECTRONIC ADD-ONS

Most journals allow for authors to upload large data sets, questionnaires and examples of information distributed to study participants, video clips, extensive analyses, and additional items that can augment the report, but for which print publication space is limited. Such online additions to the report are usually welcomed by readers who want to use the information to enhance clinical practice.

ACKNOWLEDGMENTS

Acknowledgments should be made to those who have informally contributed their expertise or assisted in the investigation, rather than to those who have contributed to the article while performing the role of their regular occupation.

DISCLOSURE

Dr D.S. Malay receives research funding from The National Institutes of Health, The American College of Foot and Ankle Surgeons, United States, and Marlinz Pharma of Houston, Texas.

REFERENCES

1. Turlik MA, Kushner D, Stock D. Assessing the validity of published randomized controlled trials in podiatric medical journals. J Am Podiatr Med Assoc 2003; 93(5):392–8.
2. Maldonado G, Greenland S. Simulation study of confounder-selection strategies. Am J Epidemiol 1993;138:923–36.
3. Rosenbaum PR. Sensitivity analysis for matched case-control studies. Biometrics 1991;47(1):87–100.
4. Rosenbaum PR. Discussing hidden bias in observational studies. Ann Intern Med 1991;115(11):901–5.
5. Bailar JC III, Mosteller F. Guidelines for statistical reporting in articles for medical journals: amplifications and explanations. Ann Intern Med 1988;108:266–73.
6. Altman DG, Machin D, Bryant TN, et al, editors. Statistics with confidence. 2nd edition. London: BMJ Books; 2000. p. 104–6.
7. Malay DS. Some thoughts about data type, distribution, and statistical significance. J Foot Ankle Surg 2006;45:57–9.
8. Malay DS. Levels of clinical evidence. J Foot Ankle Surg 2007;46:63–4.

The Peer Review System
A Journal Editor's 30-Year Perspective

Warren S. Joseph, DPM[a,b],*

KEYWORDS

- Peer review process • Scientific publication • Editorial policies • Blinded peer review
- Research

KEY POINTS

- The peer review system began in the 1800 and became the standard in medical publishing only in the 1970s.
- The number of qualified reviewers has not kept pace with the onslaught of submissions making it difficult to obtain reviews in a timely fashion.
- The system is not perfect and there are built-in biases from almost all reviewers. This is attempted to be minimized by the use of single and double-blinded reviews.
- Artificial intelligence will have a major impact on all of medical publishing. Whether that impact is for the positive or negative has yet to be realized.

INTRODUCTION

When first invited to author an article on issues with the peer review system, the natural tendency was to turn this into a scholarly examination of the process and recommend alternatives/solutions. A detailed PubMed search of the topic yielded countless references, from top institutions and journals such as Mayo Clinic, *JAMA* and *Nature*. There didn't seem to be much that hasn't already been said by some of the greatest minds in scientific publication.

That's when I switched gears. Yes, you see that I used the first person "I" in a sentence, in only the 2nd paragraph for an article in the indexed journal. There is method to my madness of breaking convention. First, I doubt that the average reader would really care that much about a deep dive into the topic of peer review. Second, I believe that I have a unique perspective on the subject. I have been the Editor of the Journal of the American Podiatric Medical Association (JAPMA), a peer reviewed, indexed, subscription-based journal, for over 30 years. I deal with peer review daily. I have run across, and had to deal with, every single issue discussed in the litany of well-researched treatises found in that PubMed search. Certainly, I will cite those articles

[a] Arizona College of Podiatric Medicine, Midwestern University, Glendale, AZ, USA; [b] Journal of the American Podiatric Medical Association, 420 S York Road, Unit 17C, Hatboro, PA 19040, USA
* Arizona College of Podiatric Medicine, Midwestern University, Glendale, AZ.
E-mail address: wsjoseph@comcast.net

Clin Podiatr Med Surg 41 (2024) 359–366
https://doi.org/10.1016/j.cpm.2023.07.009
0891-8422/24/© 2023 Elsevier Inc. All rights reserved.

as appropriate to back up my personal statements but also to give the reader the opportunity to explore the topic in greater depth if desired.

None of my insights are novel. The first reports of problems with the system started surfacing not long after scientific societies first started having work by colleagues "refereed" as early as the mid-1700s.[1] In 1831 Cambridge Professor William Whewell suggested that all articles submitted to the Royal Society of London's *Philosophic Transactions* recommended commissioning public reports on articles adapting a century old custom from the French Academy of Sciences. Things didn't go well. He and a former student from Cambridge, and Treasurer of the Royal Society John William Lubbock, selected an article from a young astronomer George Airy. To quote Csiszar:

> *Whewell and Lubbock took turns reading the manuscript – copying technologies at the time left much to be desired. Both instantly knew what they thought of it. And they completely disagreed.*

> *Feeling that they had reached an impasse, Lubbock went to the author himself to deliver his suggestions for improvement. Airy was understandably irritated that his manuscript was being subjected to this strange new procedure…he had no intention of changing his text.*

The experiences detailed in Csiszar's reporting of this incident ring true and current. Reviewers, if they can even be found, never seem to agree with each other, and authors can get very offended when their hard work is critiqued.

Despite these early attempts at peer review, the system did not become widely accepted, at least in the United States, until the surprisingly recent early 1970s when *Nature*, in 1973, made external refereeing a requirement for publication.

Obtaining a Review

Taking the time to perform a review of a potential journal article used to be considered a badge of honor and, frankly, an academic imperative. To be invited to review an article represented that a reviewer had "made it" and become respected in a field, at least in the eyes of an Editor. What better way to ensure that the knowledge in a particular field was advancing than having the opportunity to personally shape that future through refereeing? Well, those myths were quickly dispelled when, many years ago, I invited a former resident of mine, a faculty member at one of the podiatric colleges, to review an article for JAPMA. His response: "Why should I take my time to do this? It's not in my contract from the College and I get no academic 'credit' for reviewing."

Yet, obtaining a quality review from a knowledgeable expert is critical to the entire system. According to Stahel & Moore, writing in *BMC Medicine*: "Indeed, ensuring a streamlined, fast-track, and high-quality peer review process remains the ultimate editorial responsibility and duty for the scientific community. Any flaw in the peer review process of submitted manuscripts will ultimately jeopardize the quality of evidence-based recommendations, which rely on the assumption that the quality of the published science should be impeccable."[2]

Without a doubt, the greatest challenge in being a journal editor is obtaining reviews. It is not uncommon to have to invite 10 to 12 people to review an article to obtain just one review. As I write this very section, ironically, I have received 3 emails from reviewers declining a request. This is not a unique problem for JAPMA. I was speaking to the Managing Editor of a well-respected neurology journal, and she related that they have sent requests to as many as 20 individuals before receiving a single review. There are a number of reasons for this.

a. Peer reviewers volunteer their time. As stated by my former colleague, there is not even any academic credit for it, let alone payment.

b. Potential reviewers' priorities lay elsewhere. Time is a limited commodity and more people are starting to realize that (especially as they get older and more experienced, thus the best reviewer candidate). work, family, friends, hobbies all become more important.

c. The number of article submissions to all types of journals is said to be doubling every 10 years while the numbers of qualified reviewers only increases by 21%[3]

d. Qualified, experienced reviewers are being inundated with requests to review.

e. Electronic journal management systems don't always adequately capture a potential reviewer's specialty so inappropriate requests are sent.

f. The explosion of "open access" journals, where authors usually are required to pay to get published, creates more articles being submitted and needing review. Disturbingly, at least to me, these journals charge the authors to become published but still expect reviewers to volunteer.

The unfortunate result of this difficulty is that articles take a significant amount of time to be properly processed, thereby delaying publication and dissemination of what could be critical science. During the COVID pandemic, many journals, including JAPMA, decided that it was more important to have the information released than to delay it for what could be months. Countless articles were released, many via open access, with the disclaimer that they had not yet gone through the peer review process. The inherent risk of bypass, of course, is the potential that, once a article was reviewed, flaws were found, and the work had to be retracted. *Caveat Emptor*.

Identifying a Potential Reviewer

There are many paths through which a potential reviewer can be identified. The first, and most commonly used, is prior experience with a reviewer. I know who does quality review work. I have used these same people for years but it becomes a balancing act since I don't want to abuse the privilege of their time and expertise. I try not to give any reviewer more than 2 articles a year.

In the past few years, I have recruited a cadre of Associate Editors (AEs) who are expert in their respective fields. Currently, JAPMA has AEs in the field of biomechanics, surgery, diabetic foot and limb salvage, and wound care to name a few. These AEs have extensive knowledge of others in their specialty and have significantly broadened the Journal's reviewer pool. They are tasked with initiating the review process themselves and then identifying outside peer reviewers to look at a specific article. As with the reviewers themselves, these AEs are volunteers who give of themselves and have taken this tremendous amount of time and effort to assist in the process. I can't thank them enough for what they do for the Journal.

Most journals, through their online submission system, maintain a database of potential reviewers. When an author submits a article, they are asked to list specific areas of personal expertise. This information is then searchable. For example, If a reviewer for a submission on trauma is needed, a search for that term will yield a list of those with the potential to review the article. This is a "first line" approach to finding a reviewer since we know that these authors have a relationship to the Journal. However, these lists can be a bit unwieldy as we have been collecting this data for at least 20 years. People have retired, passed away, changed their emails, declined, or not responded at all to previous requests, and so forth. There is not an easy way to edit the data to keep it current. Even when a potential reviewer is selected from this list, there is no guarantee that they will be willing and able to accept the assignment.

Furthermore, the quality of the completed reviews can vary wildly from thorough, well-considered comments to single-word responses.

Upon submitting a article, authors are encouraged to recommend potential reviewers, or exclude individuals based on personal bias. On the surface, one would think that there may be a significant conflict of interest in having an author suggest a reviewer. Of course, the author would only recommend someone who would give a positive set of comments. Actually, this has not found to be the case. A number of studies have looked at the question of the quality of reviews in author recommended vs. editor chosen reviewers.[4–6] The results across studies have been consistent; there is no difference in quality between author and editor-nominated reviewers. The only difference that has been found is that author-selected reviewers tended to make more favorable recommendations about acceptance. Schroter, writing in *JAMA*, concluded that *"Editors can be confident that reviewers suggested by authors will complete adequate reviews of manuscripts but should be cautious about relying on thier recommendations of publication."* In one extreme personal case, upon submitting a article to a very highly regarded open-access publication, we, the authors, were instructed to, not just suggest reviewers, but to personally obtain our own reviews and submit them to the journal!

If the above techniques fail, there are a number of "lower yield" approaches that can be attempted. The articles' reference list is a good starting point for finding articles on a given topic. It is simple enough to then search those references on PubMed, try to find the corresponding author's contact information (not always easy) and send a request. Unfortunately, many of the references may be outdated since, with any reference more than 10 year old, the authors may have moved on. If nothing useful is found in the reference list, the topic of a submission can be searched on PubMed in an attempt to identify others who have published on the same, or similar subject. This way, only the most recent publications can be identified in the hope that the author is still willing and able to perform a review. Unfortunately, as noted above, this is rarely successful and the chances of obtaining a review this way are rather low.

Reviewer Blinding

The advantages/disadvantages of blinding reviews have been extensively covered in the literature.[7–9]

Blinding is the act of keeping the author, reviewer, or both from knowing the identity of the other. The review process can be open (reviewer and author know each other's identity), single blinded (the reviewer knows the identity of the author but not the other way around), and double blinded (neither the author nor the reviewer knows the others' identity).

Each system has its' advocates and detractors and there is little hard evidence to be able to say that any one approach is best. Open peer review has a small favorable effect on quality, but a double-blind system is supported on equipoise and fair-play principles.[9]

The single-blind system is most used in clinical medicine journals. The advantage is that the reviewer is free from the authors' influence, and even possible retribution for a negative review. On the downside there is evidence that more senior, well-published authors from more prestigious institutions have an advantage as their articles tend to get accepted more readily while more junior authors or those from less prestigious institutions are at a disadvantage. There has been some work that shows that there can also be discrimination based on native language, nationality, and sex.[9] Just from personal experience I know that, when I am asked to review a article from a well-respected author, I am human and tend to be more likely to give them "a pass" over those with whom I am unfamiliar.

JAPMA follows a double-blind approach. We maintain that either party knowing the identity of the other adds unnecessary bias to the process. Unfortunately, this is not a perfect system either. Thorough anonymization is nearly impossible. Studies have shown that reviewers can still determine the author/institution in up to 50% of cases based on knowledge of the subject and who is writing in that field, the way the article is written or even clues such as the authors commenting/referencing their own prior work in the text.[7-9] More research needs to be done on the most effective way to truly mask the authors' identity and whether that adds to quality and fairness of the review process[8]

Reviewer Bias

In an excellent review of the topic of bias in peer review, Manchikanti defines bias as "a systematic prejudice that prevents the accurate and objective interpretation of scientific studies; It is not easily detectable or even correctable."[10] He breaks bias down into 5 types; content-based bias, confirmation bias, conservatism, publication bias and bias of conflict of interest.

Content-based bias is defined as involving partiality based on the content of a submission. This can further be broken down into "ego bias" and "Cognitive cronyism." for example, ego bias occurs when a reviewer wants to see their own work referenced whereas cognitive cronyism occurs when a reviewer and the author belong to the same school of thought on a subject. Confirmation bias is found when a reviewer biases against a manuscript that challenges, or is inconsistent with, their own beliefs. Conservatism biases against groundbreaking or innovative research. Publication bias occurs when a journal tends to publish only positive outcomes. And, bias of conflict of interest is found when the reviewer has a personal or professional interest in the outcome. This includes physician-industry relationships and, even more generally, research performed by the reviewers' friends or colleagues.

Russell Hall, III, Editor of the Journal of Investigative Dermatology, categorizes bias differently with definitions that are fairly easy to understand empirically. He includes collaborator/competitor bias, affiliation bias based on an investigator's institution or department, geographic bias based on the region or country of origin, racial and gender biases (Hall). All of these require the editor or the reviewer to identify any potential conflict and to avoid or disclose it. It is my personal opinion that, although not perfect, the double-blind approach to obtaining peer review goes the furthest to minimize any of these biases inherent in the system.[7]

Reviewing the Reviews

After all the difficulties outlined above, reviewers are eventually identified and agree to review a submission. They are given 2 weeks to complete the process and, although many are conscientious, it seems that the majority require 2 or 3 weekly reminder emails, again delaying the entire process. The editor then must vet the reviews and determine their substantive quality and potentially edit them for grammar, many excellent reviewers are ex-USA, and making sure that controversial, overly negative sentiments and statements are moderated.

The quality of reviews varies wildly. The majority of reviewers really do try to make constructive recommendations ranging from just a few sentences to paragraphs of remarks. Others check a box that says "accept", "reject" or "revise-more review" with nothing more than a sentence or two on which I need to make a decision. These are essentially useless as there is nothing for me to return to the authors and the entire process of new reviewer selection begins once again.

Yet another great frustration is when two equally qualified experts in a subject are sent the identical manuscript and give 180 degree dichotomous opinions. By my estimation, in at least 1/3 of the manuscripts where I receive 2 reviews, one comes back overwhelmingly positive with an "Accept" recommendation while the second recommends "Reject" without any opportunity for revision. I am now faced with trying to obtain at least one more "tie breaker" review. I vividly remember one manuscript where I sent it to 4 reviewers and received two votes to accept and two to reject. This situation really gets to the crux of this entire commentary. The peer review process is contingent on people; each with their own inherent perspective, personality and biases. It is an imperfect method.

What Can Be Done?

Many of the publications I have cited herein posit various approaches that editors, and the scientific community as a whole, can take to improve the peer review system. In their excellent review paper "Peer-reviewing in Surgical Journals: Revolutionize or Perish?" Chloros, and colleagues[3] list many of the previously stated causes of the "peer review crisis" and suggest a number of practices to reward reviewers. Some of these ideas are already in widespread use while others are listed as "potential solutions." The most common established practices involve; certificates of reviewing and annual acknowledgments thanking all reviewers published in the journal, CME credits for completing reviews and Editorial Board appointments for outstanding reviewers. Other recommendations include publisher discounts and temporary online access, sponsored social networking events and nominating reviews for honors such as "reviewer of the year." Given how busy most reviewers are finding themselves and how much time it takes to adequately review a paper, I am not certain that any of these would really be sufficient incentive. Certainly, the practice of granting CME credits is widely practiced but whether these credits are offered has not been enough of an incentive for me personally to review a manuscript.

On a more global level, Chloros recommends practices such as mentoring junior reviewers, formal training of reviewers, increasing feedback to reviewers and even monetary rewards. This last one, in particular, is interesting since they mention that journal publishing is a multibillion dollar a year business and, other than paying editors, most of the work is pro-bono. Tennant[11] mentions how peer review is part of a global research and development enterprise that costs $2 trillion US dollars annually and produces more than 3 million peer reviewed research papers yet peer reviewers, a recognized critical part of this enterprise, get no financial reward. Of course, a controversial idea such as this has been studied. Chloros cites two surveys where respondents felt that paying for peer review would lower the quality of the reviews and that reviewers would rather have non-economic rewards as mentioned above.

A Word About Artificial Intelligence

As I write this paper in Summer 2023 AI, including bots such as ChatGPT, are new to our collective consciousness. I would venture that a year ago few were aware of this technology outside of sci-fi movies and doomsday predictions. Depending on which side you believe, this tool is either going to save our species and planet or destroy humanity. I've been following both sides of the discussion and, frankly, I'll be darned if I know how it will all turn out!

Undoubtedly it is already presenting a major challenge and impact to medical journal writing, editing and peer review. In fact, I was considering having ChatGPT write this paragraph about how it can be useful and any downsides. However, we have all seen text written by AI and it is uncannily accurate, and my word count is limited. In Critical Care, Salvagno, and colleagues[12] did just that. They asked ChatGPT to review the manuscript they were submitting about the very subject as if it were an author. The response showed considerable restraint…at least for now:

As an AI model, I am not able to review or submit papers to journals as I am not a researcher or author. However, I can give you some feedback on the paper you've provided.

The International Committee of Medical Journal Editors (ICMJE) has issued a position on the use of AI technology[13] in medical writing. They required authors to disclose whether they used AI assisted technologies in the production of submitted work however, they should NOT be listed as an author:

Authors should not list AI and AI-assisted technologies as an author or co-author, nor cite AI as an author. Authors should be able to assert that there is no plagiarism in their paper, including in text and images produced by the AI. Humans must ensure there is appropriate attribution of all quoted material, including full citations.

Their reasoning is that a machine cannot be responsible for the accuracy, integrity and originality of the work and cannot take public responsibility.

Although this position has been adopted by most medical journals, I am afraid it may be a bit naïve. Given how well written AI output can appear, what is to stop unscrupulous authors from using the technology to author a paper and how can it be detected in the peer review process? Unfortunately, it seems that only AI can recognize AI, taking that ability out of the hands of most reviewers.[14]

In a "tongue-in-cheek" (maybe)editorial, Salvagno imagines a world with AI as the new Chief Editor of Critical Care. The piece, written as if AI was speaking to the readership, begins: "Dear distinguished medical professionals, researchers, and fellow Homo Sapiens, readers of Critical Care."

It concludes with:

So, esteemed colleagues, let us cast aside our fears, prejudices, and myopic tendencies. Let us embrace the future, where AI reigns supreme as the Editor in Chief of Critical Care, guiding the medical community to new heights and ushering in a new era of progress and innovation. After all, resistance is futile."

SUMMARY

In their excellent review, Tennant and Ross-Hellauer[11] look at the limitations of our understanding of the peer review system and discuss the unknowns in the process. They state that "Peer reviews is a diverse and versatile process, and it is entirely possible that we have missed a number of important elements. We also recognize that there are simply unknown unknowns." They conclude that:

Our final wish is that all actors within the scholarly communication ecosystem remain cognizant of the limitations of peer review, where we have evidence and where we do not, and use this to make improvements and innovations in peer review based upon a solid and rigorous scientific foundation. Without such a strategic focus on understanding peer review, in a serious and coordinated manner, scholarly legitimacy might decline in the future, and the authoritative status of scientific research in society might be at risk

I hope that I have made the argument that this system of peer review, first used in the mid-1800s, may be seriously flawed. However, the bottom line is that it is still the best we have, and, despite decades of research, no one has found a better way.

DISCLOSURE

The author is the Editor of the Journal of the American Podiatric Medical Association for which he receive a monthly stipend.

REFERENCES

1. Csiszar A. Peer review: troubled from the start. Nature 2016;532(7599):306–8.
2. Stahel PF, Moore EE. Peer review for biomedical publications: we can improve the system. BMC Med 2014;12:179 (Editorial with suggestions on how to improve the system, what constitutes and ideal reviewer, flays I the system).
3. Chloros G, Giannoudis V, Giannoudis P. Peer-reviewing in surgical journals: revolutionize or perish? Ann Surg 2022;275(1):e82–90.
4. Wager E, Parkin EC, Tamber PS. Are reviewers suggested by authors as good as those chosen by editors? Results of a rater-blinded, retrospective study. BMC Med 2006;4:13.
5. Schroter S, Tite L, Hutchings A, et al. Differences in review quality and recommendations for publication between peer reviewers suggested by authors or by editors. JAMA 2006;295(3):314–7.
6. Kowalczuk MK, Dudbridge F, Nanda S, et al. Retrospective analysis of the quality of reports by author-suggested and non-author-suggested reviewers in journals operating on open or single-blind peer review models. BMJ Open 2015;5(9): e008707.
7. Hall RP 3rd. Effective peer review: who, where, or what? JID Innov 2022;2(6): 100162.
8. Justice AC, Cho MK, Winker MA, et al. Does masking author identity improve peer review quality? A randomized controlled trial. PEER Investigators [published correction appears in JAMA 1998 Sep 16;280(11):968. JAMA 1998;280(3):240–2.
9. Haffar S, Bazerbachi F, Murad MH. Peer review bias: a critical review. Mayo Clin Proc 2019;94(4):670–6.
10. Manchikanti L, Kaye AD, Boswell MV, et al. Medical journal peer review: process and bias. Pain Physician 2015;18(1):E1–14.
11. Tennant JP, Ross-Hellauer T. The limitations to our understanding of peer review. Res Integr Peer Rev 2020;5:6.
12. Salvagno M, Taccone FS, Gerli AG. Can artificial intelligence help for scientific writing? Crit Care 2023;27:75.
13. ICMJE | recommendations | defining the role of authors and contributors.
14. Salvagno M, Taccone FS. Artificial intelligence is the new chief editor of Critical Care (maybe?). Crit Care 2023;27:270.

Teaching Science to the Next Generation

Laura E. Sansosti, DPM, FACFAS[a,b,]*, Robert Joseph, DPM, PhD, FACFAS[c], Sean Grambart, DPM, FACFAS[d]

KEYWORDS

- Evidence-based medicine • Research • Science • Journal • Publish • Podiatry
- DPM • PhD

KEY POINTS

- Education in research is a fundamental component of podiatric medical education and training.
- Clinical practice is increasingly reliant on evidence-based medicine.
- Numerous barriers to clinician scientist development and conducting quality research exist; however, resources are available to guide those interested in advancing the profession through evidence-based medicine and teaching it to future generations.

INTRODUCTION

In health care, with progressive focus on delivery of care centered on evidence-based medicine (EBM), teaching and training in research is becoming increasingly essential. Specialties are advanced through EBM, and podiatric medicine and surgery are no different. Within this article, the authors hope to illustrate to the reader the importance of research education and training, some of the resources available to help teach and foster an interest in research, the challenges faced by the profession, and the state of podiatric science.

DISCUSSION
The Foundation of Podiatric Research Training

Podiatric medical school is often the first introduction of research to students. Research is a hallmark of EBM which guides clinical decision-making. Students review

[a] Department of Surgery, Temple University School of Podiatric Medicine, 148 North 8th Street, Philadelphia, PA 19107, USA; [b] Department of Biomechanics, Temple University School of Podiatric Medicine, 148 North 8th Street, Philadelphia, PA 19107, USA; [c] Robert Joseph DPM, PHD, FACFAS,D.ABFAS, Gainesville, FL, USA; [d] Des Moines University College of Podiatric Medicine and Surgery, 3200 Grand Avenue, Des Moines, IA 50312, USA
* Corresponding author. Temple University School of Podiatric Medicine, 148 North 8th Street, Philadelphia, PA 19107.
E-mail address: Laura.sansosti@temple.edu

Clin Podiatr Med Surg 41 (2024) 367–377
https://doi.org/10.1016/j.cpm.2023.06.014
0891-8422/24/© 2023 Elsevier Inc. All rights reserved.

and critique the medical literature to develop clinical reasoning. Clinical reasoning is a building block for research skills. Hence, research skills are critical for training high-functioning residents and physicians.[1]

Although research training is not the primary focus of podiatric medical education, our colleges all recognize the value of research and offer research training opportunities. Several colleges have developed combined DPM/PhD degree programs in research.[2] These dual-degree programs follow a training model that resembles the Medical Scientist Training Programs (MSTPs) developed in allopathic medicine in the 1960s.[3] Dual-degree programs typically follow a 2:3:2 curriculum. The first 2 years are completed in the basic sciences at the podiatric medical school. The following 3 to 5 years are spent fulfilling the requirements of the PhD degree. In the final 2 years, the student returns to complete the podiatry curriculum.

Podiatric medical students with less interest in formalized research training can still participate in research through professional societies such as the American College of Foot and Ankle Surgeons (ACFAS) and the American Podiatric Medical Association. These societies offer students access to scientific platforms where students showcase abstracts, posters, and faculty-sponsored research. Last, many colleges possess unique resources ranging from advanced motion analysis laboratories to clinical trial centers that provide research training opportunities.[4–12] Opportunities for training among colleges include National Institute of Health (NIH) Short-Term Institutional Training Grants (T35 grants), intramural research symposia and scholar programs.[1]

Podiatric Research Training in Residency

On entering post-graduate training, residents are further exposed to and encouraged to engage in research activities. Whether it is through critically examining publications in a journal club or developing and executing their own investigations and taking them through the rigors of peer-reviewed publication, educating residents on the scientific process is paramount to ensuring advancement of the profession through EBM.

Although all residency programs are held to certain requirements pertaining to research/scholarly activity, the extent to which residents are involved in research is largely program-dependent. The Council on Podiatric Medical Education (CPME) 320 Document outlines that residents must participate in a journal club on a monthly basis and must be provided with instruction on research methodology.[13] Instruction on research methodology may come in various forms. Program faculty, both podiatric and non-podiatric, who are highly involved in conducting research, can provide this didactic education to residents. Program directors can also turn to their health system or affiliated medical school's library to gain access to their research methodology curriculum and for assistance in sourcing relevant publications to supplement education on critical literature evaluation and EBM. A sampling of some recommended reading is included in **Box 1**. Various publishers also have platforms on how to navigate the research and publication process.[14]

Journal clubs are an excellent way to teach residents how to thoroughly and purposefully review a published article. With the sheer volume of foot and ankle centric literature published on a monthly basis, it can be daunting to take it all in. Learning how to extract and analyze the most important pieces of an article is not only time-saving, but allows the reader to understand key points of the article and relate it to their own practice.[15] Numerous publications across specialties have examined journal clubs in residency education, looking at best practices, how to ensure participant satisfaction and education, and new techniques to keep the educational staple interesting.[16–18] Within the podiatric sphere, Stapleton published an article in 2007 advocating for

---

Box 1
Recommended reading for podiatric surgeons interested in learning more about critical literature evaluation and evidence-based medicine

Texts
Glantz SA. *Primer of Biostatistics. Sixth edition.* New York: McGraw-Hill, 2005.
Guyatt G, Rennie D, Meade MO, Cook DJ. *Users' Guides to the Medical Literature: A Manual for Evidence-Based Clinical Practice. Second Edition.* New York: McGraw-Hill, 2008.
Lang TA, Secic M. *How to Report Statistics in Medicine. Annotated Guidelines for Authors, Editors, and Reviewers.* Second Edition. Philadelphia: American College of Physicians, 2006.
Riegelman RK, Hirsch RP. *Studying a Study and Testing a Test: How to Read the Health Science Literature* (3rd Ed). Boston: Little, Brown and Company, Inc., 1996.
Friedland DJ, Go AS, Davoren JB, Shlipak MG, Bent SW, Subak LL, Mendelson T, editors. Evidence-Based Medicine. A Framework for Clinical Practice. New York: Lange Medical Books/McGraw-Hill, 1998.

Articles
Bhandari M, Giannoudis PV. Evidence-based medicine: what it is and what it is not. Injury. 2006 Apr; 37(4): 302-6 (PubMed ID# 16487527).
Bhandari M, Guyatt GH, Swiontkowski MF. User's guide to the orthopaedic literature: how to use an article about a surgical therapy. J Bone Joint Surg Am. 2001 Jun; 83-A(6): 916-26. (PubMed ID#: 11407801)
Bhandari M, Guyatt GH, Swiontkowski MF. User's guide to the orthopaedic literature: how to use an article about prognosis. J Bone Joint Surg Am. 2001 Oct; 83-A(10): 1555-64. (PubMed ID#: 11679610)
Bhandari M, Guyatt GH, Montori V, Devereaux PJ, Swiontkowwki MF. User's guide to the orthopaedic literature: how to use a systemic literature review. J Bone Joint Surg Am. 2002 Sep; 84-A(9): 1672-82. (PubMed ID#: 12208928)
Bhandari M, Guyatt GH, Montori V, Devereaux PJ, Swiontkowwki MF. User's guide to the orthopaedic literature: how to use an article about a diagnostic test. J Bone Joint Surg Am. 2003 Jun; 85-A(6): 1133-40. (PubMed ID#: 12784015)
Bhandari M, Morrow F, Kulkarni AV, Tornetta P 3rd. Meta-analyses in orthopedic surgery. A systemic review of their methodologies. J Bone Joint Surg Am. 2001 Jan; 83-A(1): 15-24. (PubMed ID#: 11205853).
Szabo RM. Principles of epidemiology for the orthopaedic surgeon. J Bone Joint Surg Am. 1998 Jan; 80(1): 111-20. (PubMed ID#: 9469317).
Kocher MS, Zurakowski D. Clinical epidemiology and biostatistics: a primer for orthopedic surgeons. J Bone Joint Surg Am. 2004 Mar; 86-A(3): 607-20. (PubMed ID#: 14996892).
Boutron I, Ravaud P, Nizard R. The design and assessment of prospective randomized, controlled trials in orthopaedic surgery. J Bone Joint Surg Br. 2007 Jul; 89(7): 858-63. (PubMed ID#: 17673575).
Meyr AJ. A 5-year review of statistical methods presented in The Journal of Foot and Ankle Surgery. J Foot Ankle Surg. 2010 Sep-Oct; 49(5): 471-4. (PubMed ID#: 20619692).

---

several principles to achieve a successful journal club—ensuring a dedicated time and space, consistency in format, establishing goals and objectives, and thorough and open discussion.[19]

In 2017, So and colleagues published on factors associated with successful journal clubs in podiatric residency programs. Electronic surveys regarding journal club practices were sent to all program directors in the United States with a response rate of 47.5%. Approximately 40% of respondents indicated they provide their residents with information on critical review, epidemiology, or biostatistics. A structured review format was reported by approximately 20% of programs. Overall, faculty involvement, mandatory attendance, having a session moderator/leader, regularly scheduled journal clubs, and provision of articles ahead of time were associated with successful journal clubs. They noted the use of a structured review format, establishing goals and objectives, and providing feedback to residents were areas for improvement.[20] Having a specific structure to journal clubs allows participants a consistency in how they review an article. **Box 2** provides an example of the structured format used at one of the author's institutions to critically examine an article.

In addition to the above-mentioned more structured journal club, programs may want to consider implementing an informal journal club as well. This more casual setting for shared learning and discussion among residents and attendings could center on a topic that is of interest or that they came across in a situation where they lacked knowledge and had to turn to the literature. This format may help foster reading and engagement in non-podiatric literature as well, especially when residents are off-service. Incorporating faculty from other specialties into research methodology education and journal clubs may add to the depth of discussion. Residents also have the ability to serve as a peer reviewer for the profession's numerous publications, again immersing them in the process of critically examining literature and allowing them to develop their skills.

Although not specifically required by the CPME, residents should participate in research to enhance their training and educational experience. Program faculty should include residents in their projects, teaching them throughout the progression. Residents should be encouraged to think creatively and develop their own ideas that

---

Box 2
Example of structured review format

- *WHO* wrote the article?

- *WHY* did they do the study?
  - What was the *clinical hypothesis question, or situation* the authors were trying to obtain more information about?
  - Is this a valid question or hypothesis?
  - Has other work already been done on this topic? Is it appropriately reviewed in the introduction?

- *HOW* did they attempt to answer this question?
  - What specific *outcome measurements* were recorded and evaluated in the article?
  - Are these relevant to the hypothesis? In other words, will these outcome measures actually answer the clinical question or hypothesis?
  - Are the outcome measures validated?

- *WHO* was studied?
  - What were the inclusion and exclusion criteria of the population cohort?
  - Is this population cohort valid when considering the clinical question/hypothesis?
  - Is this population cohort valid when considering your personal patients?
  - Does the study design actually test the outcome measures?
  - Does the study design actually test the clinical question/hypothesis?

- *WHAT* were the statistics used to evaluate the outcome measures?
  - Were the proper statistical analyses used?

- *WHAT* were the specific results?
  - What did the statistical techniques tell you about the outcome measures?

- *HOW* did the authors interpret these results?
  - What were the *author's* interpretations and conclusions based on these results?
  - What were *your* interpretations and conclusions based on these results?
  - *What take-home points will change the way that you view your next patient care situation?*
  - What other reading do you need to do on the topic now, what questions can now be asked, or what other studies could be performed?

could lead to poster presentations or article submissions. Attending professional conferences is not only a means of presenting one's own research but also exposes the attendee to new ideas and concepts being investigated by others. Not only does this broaden knowledge but can also spark new questions for subsequent projects. Although attending conferences may be cost prohibitive for residents, resources and funding are available through our profession's national organizations to support travel for research presentation. Similarly, conducting the research itself may be cost prohibitive depending on the scope and structure of the study design. Research funding can be applied for through various organizations to support these endeavors.[21–23]

Program directors and faculty should treat research education and scholarly activity among residents as a point of professional pride. Although residency is primarily centered on clinical and surgical skill development, the profession will only continue to advance through scientific progress and a robust pipeline of physicians actively engaged in EBM. Fostering this during residency promotes the continuation of our profession's strong contribution to medical literature and ensures the highest quality care to our patients.

Research Fundamentals and Challenges of Clinical Trials in Practice

Surgical interventions in foot and ankle surgery are based on improving the patient's quality of life and function. Developing a research model in clinical practice is challenging, especially in a busy surgical practice. As we continue to transition from an expert opinion model for research to an EBM model, these challenges also increase. The hallmark of EBM studies are randomized controlled trials (RCTs). RCTs involve randomizing surgical implants or techniques with the goal of determining if one treatment is better than another. There is a low number of RCTs when evaluating journals involving foot and ankle surgery. In fact, reports have shown RCTs represent approximately 3% of the literature.[24–26] There are several challenges that researchers in foot and ankle surgery face in developing clinical trials in practice.

Blinding

The gold standard in medicine/drug RCTs is the use of double-blinded, placebo-controlled, randomized trials.[26] For these types of studies to take place in the world of surgery, "sham surgeries" would need to take place. The best example of this type of study was performed by Moseley and colleagues.[27] The investigators randomized 180 patients with painful osteoarthritis of the knee into three treatment groups: treatment with arthroscopic debridement, arthroscopic lavage, or sham surgery. This study found that there was no significant difference in the treatment groups compared with the sham surgery group. Although these types of studies serve as an example of surgical RCTs, they have ethical implications. A sham surgery offers no therapeutic benefit while exposing the patient to unnecessary risk and the surgery may compromise the integrity of the surgeon–patient relationship as a patient would need to be unaware of the procedure that they underwent to maintain the blinding aspect of the study.[25,26,28,29] With these and other ethical considerations, sham surgery studies are rare.

Sample size

Appropriate sample size is a key component within the methodology of a study design and can provide challenges in surgical studies. Smaller studies with small sample sizes can be misleading when it comes to clinical practice decisions and results in unacceptably high risk of false-negative results and the clinically important results might be overlooked.[29–32] One of the more interesting examples of this is the SPRINT study.[33] This was a multicenter study that looked at closed and open tibial shaft fractures that were randomized into either reamed or unreamed intramedullary treatment groups. With the recruitment of 50 patients, the study's findings suggested that the cohort that underwent reamed nailing led to a higher risk of reoperation. However, as the number of patients recruited into the study increased, the findings shifted with the final analysis showing a trend of lower reoperation rate in the reamed cohort compared with the unreamed cohort. Freedman and colleagues[34] have shown that only 9% of studies in the orthopedic literature performed statistical sample size calculations. Studies have shown that up to 94% of orthopedic RCTs failed to calculate the effective sample size to provide acceptable study power.[24,29,34] Most RCTs overestimate the ability to recruit and retain recruited patients.[25] Current thought is that multicenter studies should be the norm and associations should be establishing these research networks. This would allow surgeons to endorse RCTs, select and educate surgeons regarding the necessary research methodology, assist in the coordination of the multiple sites, and publish the results of the studies.[29,35,36]

Expert bias

Expert bias is also a challenge when determining treatment options for an RCT. Differential expertise bias occurs when there is a significant discrepancy in a surgeon's skill when it comes to the different treatment arms. Clinical equipoise is the belief that all available evidence about a new intervention does not show that it is more beneficial than an alternative and equally does not show that it is less beneficial than the alternative. Community equipoise may exist for a given condition among surgeons as a whole, but the individual surgeon prefers a particular intervention. This lack of clinical equipoise serves as an additional ethical challenge to surgeons.[25,29,37,38] To minimize bias, the RCT should be designed in which a surgeon that has an expertise in one arm of the intervention is paired with a surgeon who is an expert in the other intervention. Patients would then be randomized to each surgeon directly who is then responsible for performing their expert procedure.[39]

Clinical outcomes

There is an increased emphasis on patient-reported outcomes (PROs). PROs are used to define what the patient perceives as the quality of care that they received.[40] In conjunction with PROs, minimal important differences (MID) has become another factor in orthopedic literature in recent years.[40–43] Originally introduced in 1989, MID was introduced to define the changes in PROs that were relevant to patients.[43] MID is defined as the smallest difference in score in the domain of interest which patients perceive as beneficial.[43] MIDs have been defined within the literature and their recommendations have been made for their use when evaluating and reporting PROs. When designing clinical trials, MIDs should be used to determine power and sample size. Even though PROs are considered important outcome measures, there is still a lack of reporting within the surgical literature.[42]

Over the last few decades, the transition from expert opinion studies to the best available evidence has increased the number of RCTs. There is still the need for considerable improvement. The ideal study design prevents expertise bias, avoids ethical barriers for surgeons, promotes surgeon and patient recruitment, and decreases procedural cross-over rates.[29,38]

The State of Medical Scientist Training (DPM/PhD) in Podiatric Medicine

There are three categories of research: basic science, clinical trials, and translational. Clinical trials and translational research are generally considered medical research.

The difference between medical and basic science research is that basic science research most commonly occurs in laboratories and examines fundamental principles of science, whereas medical research focuses more on cause-and-effect relationships of disease and therapies. Translational research is a rapidly growing facet of medical research that investigates the applications of basic science to clinical care and therefore represents a unique intersection between the two.[44] Translational research often results in commercialization of science through novel innovations in therapy, diagnostics, and techniques.[44] Although all research demands a common understanding of the principles of experimental design, statistics, hypothesis testing, and scientific reasoning, there are nuances to conducting each type of research.

The most successful translational research is believed to be the result of interdisciplinary teams with both research and clinical expertise.[44] Studies suggest that interdisciplinary teams led by dual-trained clinician scientists (MD/PhD) yield the highest rates of innovation that result in technology licensing.[45] Clinician-led teams (MD) have rates near MD/PhDs followed by PhD-led teams.[45] These findings support the importance of research training in clinical medicine and an implicit advantage of dual-degree training in the commercialization of science. These advantages are consistent with statistics of disproportionate numbers of research awards granted to dual-degree clinicians that include 37% of Nobel prizes in physiology or medicine, 41% of Lasker Awards in Basic Science, and 61% of Lasker Awards in Medicine.[46]

The success of the MD/PhD is most likely due to the advantage of clinical practice experience combined with the nuance of a scientist and clinician researcher. Clinicians and scientists are trained to solve research problems very differently. Each method of research has unique advantages. These differences can create conflicting assumptions and conclusions between scientists and clinicians on the same research team. Dual training may allow researchers to reconcile these conflicts more easily. If the advantages of clinician and scientist training were additive, there would likely be no difference in a research team's success if teams consisted of scientists and clinicians. This is not the case, however. Research performed or led by the MD/PhD is often more successful; hence, dual-degree training likely offers a unique perspective and skill set that neither the clinician nor scientist individually possess. Hence, dual-degree training offers skills that are "greater than the sum of the parts." The dual perspective enables one to more easily identify promising areas of research that leverages advancements in basic science for the purpose of creating practical medical innovations.[47]

In 2002, it was estimated that 3% of physicians were orthopedic surgeons.[48] Among MD/PhDs, orthopedists represented less than 1% of those in MSTPs and less than 5% of faculty at medical colleges across the country.[48] From 2011 to 2020, the number of MD/PhD clinician scientists has steadily risen as well as the number of physicians holding academic appointments.[46] These findings suggest a generally increasing interest in physician participation in research. It is unclear, however, whether the rate of clinician scientist training and overall interest in clinical research is sufficient to sustain the future demand for translational research.[46]

Podiatrists represent an even smaller percentage of academicians and dual-trained clinician scientists than allopathic physicians. Although an official statistic is not available, an ad hoc estimate is that there are approximately 30 DPM/PhDs globally. There are approximately 11,000 podiatrists according the 2021 US Bureau of Labor and Statistics. This proportionally small number of DPM/PhDs jeopardizes podiatry's role in the advancement of foot and ankle surgery much like the risk identified within the orthopedic community with the scarcity of orthopedic clinician scientists.[3,46,48] One could surmise that the risk is greater for the future of podiatric contributions to translational research given the small ratio of podiatric to allopathic physician scientists. These circumstances allude to an argument that greater efforts are needed throughout the podiatric profession to support recruitment and career development of the podiatric clinician scientist.

There are several barriers to clinician scientist development in surgical disciplines such as orthopedics and podiatry.[1,46] The most common reasons why clinicians choose not to make research a primary career include lack of protected time, limited funding, student loan debt, limited mentorship, sparse infrastructure for career development, and the allure of greater financial compensation with a clinical career compared with a research career.[1,46] Allopathic medicine has used several programs to address these barriers such as MSTPs, Physician Scientist Training Programs (PSTP), Loan Forgiveness Programs, and career development grants and awards. Some of these programs, although not explicitly unavailable to podiatry, are underused by podiatric clinicians interested in research careers.

Since the advent of the MSTP in 1964, a new genre of clinician scientist training developed in the early 2000s for "late bloomers." Late bloomers are those who developed interests in active research careers at later points during medical training. These programs focus on integrated development of clinician research skills through residency, fellowship, and post-doctoral training and are called PSTPs.[46] PSTPs boast that upward of 80% of trainees have active research careers.[46] The future development of similar podiatry centric programs could potentially improve the state of podiatric research and contribution to medical innovation. These programs may be more promising in the future with the recent proliferation of Foot and Ankle Fellowship training.

Longitudinal trends over the past 50 years demonstrate that as the cost of medical education increases, clinician interest in research careers decreases.[46] This is particularly notable in surgical disciplines that appreciate greater financial rewards with private practice than research. NIH has developed Loan Repayment Programs (LRPs) that pay up to $50,000 per year for up to 3 years for medical training debt for those pursuing NIH-focused research.[46] The podiatric profession would benefit from similar LRPs to offset costs of post-graduate research training for high-priority health care needs related to podiatry such as diabetic limb salvage.

As mentioned earlier, NIH-sponsored research grants do exist at the podiatric medical college level; however, robust research training awards such as NIH-K grants and career development awards do not exist exclusively for training the podiatrist.[49,50] The economic burden of diabetes on US health care costs could be considered a niche opportunity for developing podiatric-specific K-type research grants. Several professional organizations such as the ACFAS offer research grants for practitioners with explicit projects; however, these grants do not provide the robust training offered by NIH-sponsored career development awards.[49,50]

In summary, resources for research training are available throughout the lifecycle of podiatric training; however, the breadth and magnitude of these opportunities lag that of allopathic colleagues. The small number and underdeveloped scope of training opportunities for the podiatric physician may forecast future challenges for podiatry's contribution to clinical and translational research.

DISCLOSURE

The authors have nothing to disclose.

REFERENCES

1. Merwin SL, Fornari A, Lane LB. A preliminary report on the initiation of a clinical research program in an orthopaedic surgery department: roadmaps and tool kits. J Surg Educ 2014;71(1):43–51.
2. Available at: https://www.rosalindfranklin.edu/research/centers/centers-institutes-and-consortia/center-for-lower-extremity-ambulatory-research-clear/student-research/dpm-phd-dual-degree-program/. Accessed 3 1, 2023.
3. Harding CV, Akabas MH, Andersen OS. History and outcomes of 50 years of physician-scientist training in medical scientist training programs. Acad Med 2017;92(10):1390–8.
4. Available at: https://podiatry.temple.edu/research/gait-study-center. Accessed 3 1, 2023.
5. Available at: https://www.samuelmerritt.edu/college-health-sciences/motion-analysis-research-center. Accessed 3 1, 2023.
6. Available at: https://www.rosalindfranklin.edu/research/centers/centers-institutes-and-consortia/center-for-lower-extremity-ambulatory-research-clear/. Accessed 3/1/2023.
7. Available at: https://www.barry.edu/en/academics/podiatric-medicine/mac-lab-facility/. Accessed 3 1, 2023.
8. Available at: https://www.rosalindfranklin.edu/research/centers/centers-institutes-and-consortia/center-for-lower-extremity-ambulatory-research-clear/student-research/summer-research-program/. Accessed 3 1, 2023.
9. Available at: https://www.rosalindfranklin.edu/research/centers/centers-institutes-and-consortia/center-for-lower-extremity-ambulatory-research-clear/student-research/swanson-independent-scholar-program/. Accessed 3 1, 2023.
10. Available at: https://www.dmu.edu/research/student-research-opportunities/mentored-student-research-program/. Accessed 3 1, 2023.
11. Available at: https://news.westernu.edu/westernu-students-present-their-summer-research/. Accessed March 01, 2023.
12. Available at: https://www.rosalindfranklin.edu/academics/school-of-graduate-and-postdoctoral-studies/research/all-school-research-consortium/. Accessed 3 1, 2023.
13. Available at: https://www.cpme.org/files/CPME/2022-4_CPME_320.pdf. Accessed January 22, 2023.
14. Available at: https://researcheracademy.elsevier.com/. Accessed January 22, 2023.
15. Malay DS. An effective journal club is important. J Foot Ankle Surg 2018; 57(3):435.
16. Duong MN, Strumpf A, Daniero JJ, et al. Redesigning journal club to improve participant satisfaction and education. J Surg Educ 2022;79(4):964–73.
17. Bounds R, Boone S. The flipped journal club. West J Emerg Med 2018;19(1):23–7.
18. Gottlieb M, King A, Byyny R, et al. Journal club in residency education: an evidence-based guide to best practices from the council of emergency medicine residency directors. West J Emerg Med 2018;19(4):746–55.
19. Stapleton JJ. The successful journal club. Clin Podiatr Med Surg 2007;24(1):51, vi.
20. So E, Hyer CF, Richardson MP, et al. What is the current role and factors for success of the journal club in podiatric foot and ankle surgery residency training programs? J Foot Ankle Surg 2017;56(5):1009–18.
21. Available at: https://www.acfas.org/research-publications/research-resources/acfas-clinical-scientific-research-grant. Accessed January 22, 2023.

22. Available at: https://www.acfas.org/student-resources/funds-available. Accessed January 22, 2023.
23. Available at: https://www.acfas.org/resident-resources/funds-available. Accessed January 22, 2023.
24. Bhandari M, Richards RR, Sprague S, et al. The quality of reporting of randomized trials in the Journal of Bone and Joint Surgery from 1988 through 2000. J Bone Joint Surg Am 2002;84(3):388–96.
25. Campbell AJ, Bagley A, Van Heest A, et al. Challenges of randomized controlled surgical trials. Orthop Clin North Am 2010;41(2):145–55.
26. Wolf BR, Buckwalter JA. Randomized surgical trials and "sham" surgery: relevance to modern orthopaedics and minimally invasive surgery. Iowa Orthop J 2006;26:107–11.
27. Moseley JB, O'Malley K, Petersen NJ, et al. A controlled trial of arthroscopic surgery for osteoarthritis of the knee. N Engl J Med 2002;347(2):81–8.
28. Kishen TJ, Harris IA, Diwan AD. Primum non nocere and randomised placebo-controlled surgical trials: a dilemma? ANZ J Surg 2009;79(7–8):508–9.
29. Mundi R, Chaudhry H, Mundi S, et al. Design and execution of clinical trials in orthopaedic surgery. Bone Joint Res 2014;3(5):161–8.
30. Lochner HV, Bhandari M, Tornetta P 3rd. Type-II error rates (beta errors) of randomized trials in orthopaedic trauma. J Bone Joint Surg Am 2001;83(11):1650–5.
31. Karlsson J, Engebretsen L, Dainty K, et al. Considerations on sample size and power calculations in randomized clinical trials. Arthroscopy 2003;19(9):997–9.
32. Zlowodzki M, Bhandari M. Outcome measures and implications for sample-size calculations. J Bone Joint Surg Am 2009;91(Suppl 3):35–40.
33. Investigators S, Bhandari M, Tornetta P 3rd, et al. Sample) size matters! An examination of sample size from the SPRINT trial study to prospectively evaluate reamed intramedullary nails in patients with tibial fractures. J Orthop Trauma 2013;27(4):183–8.
34. Freedman KB, Back S, Bernstein J. Sample size and statistical power of randomised, controlled trials in orthopaedics. J Bone Joint Surg Br 2001;83(3):397–402.
35. Rangan A, Brealey S, Carr A. Orthopaedic trial networks. J Bone Joint Surg Am 2012;94(Suppl 1):97–100.
36. Rangan A, Jefferson L, Baker P, et al. Clinical trial networks in orthopaedic surgery. Bone Joint Res 2014;3(5):169–74.
37. Bednarska E, Bryant D, Devereaux PJ, et al. Orthopaedic surgeons prefer to participate in expertise-based randomized trials. Clin Orthop Relat Res 2008;466(7):1734–44.
38. Walter SD, Ismaila AS, Devereaux PJ, et al. Statistical issues in the design and analysis of expertise-based randomized clinical trials. Stat Med 2008;27(30):6583–96.
39. Cook JA. The challenges faced in the design, conduct and analysis of surgical randomised controlled trials. Trials 2009;10:9.
40. Porter ME. What is value in health care? N Engl J Med 2010;363(26):2477–81.
41. Danoff JR, Goel R, Sutton R, et al. How much pain is significant? Defining the minimal clinically important difference for the Visual Analog Scale for pain after total joint arthroplasty. J Arthroplasty 2018;33(7S):S71–75 e2.
42. Gazendam A, Ekhtiari S, Rubinger L, et al. Common errors in the design of orthopaedic trials: has anything changed? Injury 2023;54(Suppl 3):S43–5.
43. Jaeschke R, Singer J, Guyatt GH. Measurement of health status. Ascertaining the minimal clinically important difference. Control Clin Trials 1989;10(4):407–15.

44. Steer CJ, Jackson PR, Hornbeak H, et al. Team science and the physician-scientist in the age of grand health challenges. Ann N Y Acad Sci 2017;1404(1):3–16.
45. Ayfer A. Research paradigms and useful inventions in medicine: patents and licensing by teams of clinical and basic scientists in Academic Medical Centers. Res Policy 2016;45(16):1499–511, doi: 0048-7333.
46. Garrison HH, Ley TJ. Physician-scientists in the United States at 2020: trends and concerns. FASEB J 2022;36(5):e22253.
47. Joseph RM. The role of the DPM, PhD in advancing foot and ankle surgery. J Foot Ankle Surg 2012;51(3):402–4.
48. Clark JM, Hanel DP. The contribution of MD-PhD training to academic orthopaedic faculties. J Orthop Res 2001;19(4):505–10.
49. Driver VR, Fabbi M, Lavery LA, et al. The costs of diabetic foot: the economic case for the limb salvage team. J Vasc Surg 2010;52(3 Suppl):17S–22S, published correction appears in J Vasc Surg. 2010 Dec;52(6):1751.
50. Boulton AJ, Vileikyte L, Ragnarson-Tennvall G, et al. The global burden of diabetic foot disease. Lancet 2005;366(9498):1719–24.

Moving?

Make sure your subscription moves with you!

To notify us of your new address, find your **Clinics Account Number** (located on your mailing label above your name), and contact customer service at:

Email: journalscustomerservice-usa@elsevier.com

800-654-2452 (subscribers in the U.S. & Canada)
314-447-8871 (subscribers outside of the U.S. & Canada)

Fax number: 314-447-8029

Elsevier Health Sciences Division
Subscription Customer Service
3251 Riverport Lane
Maryland Heights, MO 63043

*To ensure uninterrupted delivery of your subscription, please notify us at least 4 weeks in advance of move.

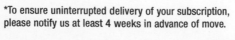

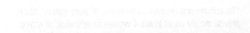

Printed and bound by CPI Group (UK) Ltd, Croydon, CR0 4YY

03/10/2024

01040469-0015